Official Journal of the

eau
European Association of Urology

EORTC
European Organization for Research and Treatment of Cancer – Genito-Urinary Group

ESUOE
European Society for Urological Oncology and Endocrinology

European Urology

KARGER

Printed in Switzerland on acid-free paper by Druckerei Schüler AG, Biel

Appears monthly: 2 volumes per year (12 issues)

Guidelines for Authors

European Urology

Submission

Only original papers written in English are considered and should be sent to:

Prof. C.C. Schulman
S. Karger AG
Editorial Office European Urology
P.O. Box
CH–4009 Basel (Switzerland)
Telephone +41 61 306 1358
Fax +41 61 306 1434
E-mail e.brogli@karger.ch

Mailing address for courier deliveries only:

Allschwilerstr. 10
CH–4055 Basel (Switzerland)

Manuscripts should be submitted in triplicate (with three sets of illustrations of which one is an original), typewritten double-spaced on one side of the paper, with a wide margin.

Conditions

All manuscripts are subject to editorial review. Manuscripts are received with the explicit understanding that they are not under simultaneous consideration by any other publication. Submission of an article for publication implies the transfer of the copyright from the author to the publisher upon acceptance. Accepted papers become the permanent property of 'European Urology' and may not be reproduced by any means, in whole or in part, without the written consent of the publisher. It is the author's responsibility to obtain permission to reproduce illustrations, tables, etc. from other publications.

Arrangement

Title page: The first page of each paper should indicate the title (main title underlined), the authors' names, and the institute where the work was conducted. A short title for use as running head as well as the full address of the author to whom correspondence should be sent are also required.

Full address: The exact postal address complete with postal code must be given at the bottom of the title page. Please also supply phone and fax numbers, as well as your e-mail address.

Key words: For indexing purposes, a list of 3–10 key words in English is essential.

Abstract: Each paper needs an abstract of up to 16 lines structured with subheadings as follows: Objective(s), Methods, Results, Conclusion(s).

Small type: Paragraphs which can or must be set in smaller type (case histories, test methods, etc.) should be indicated with a 'p' (petit) in the margin on the left-hand side.

Footnotes: Avoid footnotes. When essential, they are numbered consecutively and typed at the foot of the appropriate page.

Tables and illustrations: Tables and illustrations (both numbered in Arabic numerals) should be prepared on separate sheets. Tables require a heading and figures a legend, also prepared on a separate sheet. For the reproduction of illustrations, only good drawings and original photographs can be accepted; negatives or photocopies cannot be used. Due to technical reasons, figures with a screen background should not be submitted. When possible, group several illustrations on one block for reproduction (max. size 181 × 223 mm) or provide crop marks. On the back of each illustration, indicate its number, the author's name, and 'top' with a soft pencil.

Color illustrations: Up to 6 color illustrations per page can be integrated with the text at the reduced price of CHF 660.– / USD 545.00 per page. Color illustrations are reproduced at the author's expense.

References: In the text identify references by Arabic numerals [in square brackets]. Material submitted for publication but not yet accepted should be noted as 'unpublished data' and not be included in the reference list. The list of references should include only those publications which are cited in the text. Do not alphabetize; number references in the order in which they are first mentioned in the text. The surnames of the authors followed by initials should be given. There should be no punctuation other than a comma to separate the authors. Cite all authors, 'et al' is not sufficient. Abbreviate journal names according to the Index Medicus system. (Also see International Committee of Medical Journal Editors: Uniform requirements for manuscripts submitted to biomedical journals. Br Med J 1988;296:401–405.)

Examples

(a) Papers published in periodicals: Sun J, Koto H, Chung KF: Interaction of ozone and allergen challenges on bronchial responsiveness and inflammation in sensitised guinea pigs. Int Arch Allergy Immunol 1997;112:191–195.

(b) Monographs: Matthews DE, Farewell VT: Using and Understanding Medical Statistics, ed 3, revised. Basel, Karger, 1996.

(c) Edited books: Parren PWHI, Burton DR: Antibodies against HIV-1 from phage display libraries: Mapping of an immune response and progress towards antiviral immunotherapy; in Capra JD (ed): Antibody Engineering. Chem Immunol. Basel, Karger, 1997, vol 65, pp 18–56.

Further details: Authors may consult our leaflet 'Rules for the Preparation of Manuscripts', available on request from the Publisher, S. Karger AG, P.O. Box, CH–4009 Basel (Switzerland).

Rapid Communication: Manuscripts intended for rapid communication must present new findings of sufficient importance to justify their accelerated acceptance. They should follow the general arrangement of research papers with the exception that no abstract or introduction are required. The first paragraph should include the reason for the study and the main findings. They should not exceed 8 double-spaced manuscript pages in length, including figures, tables and references. Proofs are checked by the Main Editor and not sent to the author. Review will be rapid, and once accepted, the paper will be included in the next planned issue.

Galley proofs

Unless indicated otherwise, galley proofs are sent to the first-named author and should be returned with the least possible delay. Alterations made in galley proofs, other than the correction of printer's errors, are charged to the author. No page proofs are supplied.

Reprints

Order forms and a price list are sent with the galley proofs. Orders submitted after the issue is printed are subject to considerably higher prices.

KARGER

Fax + 41 61 306 12 34
E-Mail karger@karger.ch
www.karger.com

The Guidelines for Authors are available at:
www.karger.com/journals/eur/eurinst.htm

General Information

European
Urology

Publication data: 'European Urology' is published 12 times annually. Volumes 33–34 with 6 issues each appear in 1998.

Subscription rates: Subscriptions run for a full calendar year. Prices are given per volume.

Personal subscription:
Subscription + postage and handling
CHF 332.– + CHF 23.50 Europe
CHF 332.– + CHF 35.50 Overseas
USD 241.20 + USD 23.50
(Must be in the name of, billed to, and paid by an individual. Order must be marked 'personal subscription'.)

Institutional subscription:
Subscription + postage and handling
CHF 664.– + CHF 29.40 Europe
CHF 664.– + CHF 44.40 Overseas
USD 522.00 + USD 29.40

Airmail postage: CHF 24.–, USD 20.00.
(Extra per volume.)

Discount subscription prices:
European Association of Urology
European Organization for Research and Treatment of Cancer – Genito-Urinary Group
European Society for Urological Oncology and Endocrinology

Microforms: Please direct all enquiries and orders to: University Microfilms Inc.
300 North Zeeb Road, P.O. Box 1346
Ann Arbor, MI 48106-1346 (USA)

Subscription orders: Orders can be placed at agencies, bookstores, directly with the Publisher
S. Karger AG, P.O. Box,
CH–4009 Basel (Switzerland)
or with any of the following distributors:
Deutschland: S. Karger GmbH, Postfach
D–79095 Freiburg
France: Librairie Luginbühl
36, bd de Latour-Maubourg, F–75007 Paris
Great Britain, Ireland: S. Karger Publishers
58 Grove Hill Road
Tunbridge Wells, Kent TN1 1SP
USA: S. Karger Publishers, Inc.
26 West Avon Road, P.O. Box 529
Farmington, CT 06085
India, Bangladesh, Sri Lanka:
S. Karger India Subscription Agency
B–5/132 Safdarjung Enclave
New Delhi-110029
Japan: Katakura Libri, Inc.
Take 1 Bldg, 2nd Floor, 4-5-7 Yushima
Bunkyo-ku, Tokyo 113

Change of address: Both old and new address should be sent to the subscription source.

Single issues and back volumes: Information can be obtained through the Publisher.

Advertising: Correspondence and rate requests should be addressed to the Publisher.

Bibliographic indices: This journal is regularly listed in bibliographic services, including *Current Contents®*.

Copying: This journal has been registered with the Copyright Clearance Center (CCC), as indicated by the code appearing on the first page of each article.
For readers in the US, this code signals consent for copying of articles for personal or internal use, or for the personal or internal use of specific clients, provided that the stated fee is paid per copy directly to
Copyright Clearance Center Inc.
222 Rosewood Drive
Danvers, MA 01923 (USA)
A copy of the first page of the article must accompany payment. Consent does not extend to copying for general distribution, for promotion, for creating new works, or for resale. In these cases, specific written permission must be obtained from the copyright owner,
S. Karger AG,
P.O. Box, CH–4009 Basel (Switzerland).

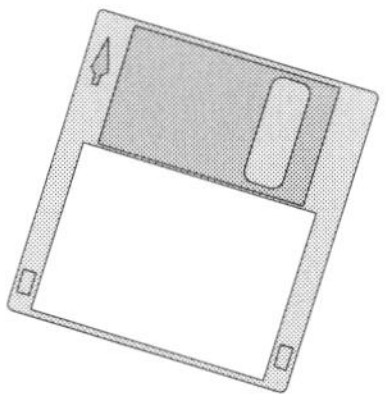

Disk Submission

A **comprehensive version** of these guidelines for the **submission of manuscripts and illustrations on disk** can be accessed online under **www.karger.com/journals/disk_mai.htm** or requested as a leaflet from the editorial department.

Please follow the general rules on style and arrangement in the **"Guidelines for Authors"** of the journal. Submit a **double-spaced printout** of your manuscript matching the file on disk exactly.

Technical Information

Store only data pertinent to this manuscript. Include your fonts (screen and printer fonts for Macintosh). For a **text only** manuscript, use a 3.5 inch disk. For **text and illustrations,** use 3.5 or 5.25 Magneto Optical Disc; CD-ROM (DOS or hybrid); iomage Zip/DOS (100 MB), or 44 MB, 88 MB or 200 MB SyQuest. Compress extensive data using ZIP format.

Data Description

Label your disk with the **title of the journal or book** for which it is submitted; a **short version** of the paper's title; your **name,** postal and e-mail address, fax and phone number; **hard and software** used, including the version; and the **complete list of the file names.** File names consist of eight characters before the dot identifying the file and three characters after the dot identifying the application.

Text and Format

The **preferred word-processing package is MS-Word.** Other commonly used PC text programs and ASCII formats are accepted.
Update your data when you revise subsequent to the reviewer's or editor's decision and mark revisions clearly. Manuscripts accepted for publication are subject to **copy editing:** changes and/or questions will be marked in the manuscript, which will be returned to you with your disk and the galley proofs for checking.
Enter your text continuously flush left. Do not use any layout functions. Do not split words at the end of a line. **Do not use indentations.** Use a blank line before and a hard return at the end of paragraphs.
Arrange headings flush left. Insert only **one space after punctuation marks.** Insert Greek letters, mathematical symbols etc. with your word-processing program. Use **boldface and italics** as well as sub- and superscript where appropriate.
Tables are part of the text and should be placed at the end of the text file. Separate the individual parts of a table by lines. Use the tabulator instead of spaces. Format operation data on one line in the same column. **Legends to illustrations are part of the text** and should also be listed at the end of the text file.

Illustrations

Store illustrations as separate files: do not embed them in your text. Export **line drawings/vector graphics** as TIF, EPS or WMF format. Use Photoshop for processing and retouching **scanned halftone images.** Save the original scan and the processed version. Export **black and white or color images** as TIF or EPS format in their anticipated size in print.
For detailed information on how to submit illustration data on disk please consult the leaflet or **www.karger.com/journals/disk_mai.htm.**

KARGER

Fax + 41 61 306 12 34
E-Mail karger@karger.ch
www.karger.com

The Journal Home Page is available at:
www.karger.com/journals/eur

KI 98 DISK

European
Urology

Proceedings of a Satellite Symposium and an Interactive Workshop held during the XIIIth EAU Congress in Barcelona, Spain, March 1998

The Management of Prostate Cancer in the Third Millennium

Editor: *Don Newling,* Amsterdam

and

Therapeutic Dilemmas in Prostate Cancer

Editor: *Frans Debruyne,* Nijmegen

12 figures and 11 tables, 1998

KARGER

Basel · Freiburg · Paris · London · New York ·
New Delhi · Bangkok · Singapore · Tokyo · Sydney

This satellite symposium and interactive workshop were sponsored by an educational grant from Zeneca Pharmaceuticals

KARGER

S. Karger
Medical and Scientific Publishers
Basel · Freiburg · Paris · London
New York · New Delhi · Bangkok
Singapore · Tokyo · Sydney

Drug Dosage
The authors and the publisher have exerted every effort to ensure that drug selection and dosage set forth in this text are in accord with current recommendations and practice at the time of publication. However, in view of ongoing research, changes in government regulations, and the constant flow of information relating to drug therapy and drug reactions, the reader is urged to check the package insert for each drug for any change in indications and dosage and for added warnings and precautions. This is particularly important when the recommended agent is a new and/or infrequently employed drug.

P.O. Box, CH–4009 Basel (Switzerland)
Printed in Switzerland on acid-free paper by
Druckerei Schüler AG, Biel
ISBN 3–8055–6799–5

Contents Vol. 34, Suppl. 3, 1998

European Urology

KARGER

Fax+ 41 61 306 12 34
E-Mail karger@karger.ch
www.karger.com

Access to full text and tables of contents,
including tentative ones for forthcoming issues:
www.karger.com/journals/eur/eurcont.htm

European Urology

D. Newling

Department of Urology, Academic Hospital Vrije University, Amsterdam, The Netherlands

Introduction

These proceedings are based on presentations made at a symposium and workshop at the XIIIth Congress of the European Association of Urology in Barcelona, Spain, 21–25 March 1998. The title of the symposium, which I was privileged and honoured to chair, was 'The management of prostate cancer in the third millennium'. The workshop was organised by Professor Frans Debruyne and is reported in the second half of this supplement.

There are several important questions in the area of prostate cancer that face both the patient and medical communities as we approach the third millennium. One of the most striking features of prostate cancer epidemiology is the large discrepancy in incidence and mortality rates between the USA and Europe. In the USA, for each patient who dies of prostate cancer a diagnosis is confirmed in eight to ten patients. In Europe this ratio is much smaller with one in four diagnosed patients dying of the disease. One possible explanation for this difference is that in the USA widespread screening programmes have led to early diagnosis and thus patients have a better prognosis, beginning treatment at an earlier stage. Another explanation might be that many patients are 'unnecessarily' treated – in other words, undergoing 'curative' treatment for diseases that do not need to be 'cured'. Certainly patients with metastatic disease have a poor prognosis with around half dying within 4 years of diagnosis. As it becomes possible to diagnose prostate cancer at an earlier stage we need to address the issue of how we determine whether patients have more or less aggressive disease in order to recommend the best treatment protocol. Dr Jack Schalken addressed this issue in his presentation and also described some of the new disease markers and therapies that are being developed with the aid of molecular medicine. Molecular research may create exciting opportunities for diagnosis and therapy of prostate cancer in the next millennium but, as Dr Schalken points out, for the possibilities to be realised there must be effective communication between the scientists and clinicians.

The ability to diagnose prostate cancer earlier also raises the subject of the cost, both in terms of money and toxicity, associated with long-term therapy. Dr Peter Iversen reassessed the role of orchidectomy and oral oestrogen therapy with the caveat that both of these treatments are associated with substantial levels of side effects. Orchidectomy may still be appropriate in some circumstances, but in the case of oestrogens, lower doses used in combination with other agents or alternative routes of administration need to be developed before the level of risk associated with this form of treatment is at an acceptable level for the patient. Quality of life issues are becoming increasingly important and the third paper in these proceedings by Professor Fritz Schröder discusses some of the quality of life benefits gained by nonsteroidal antiandrogen monotherapy. The choice of therapy will depend heavily on the priority that the patient gives to quality of life and this may depend on their life expectancy. Certainly the goal should be to improve survival and maintain quality of life for patients and in this respect monotherapy with certain nonsteroidal antiandrogens, such as bicalutamide 150 mg, looks promising.

Hormone therapy has been a big advance for the treatment of prostate cancer but we now realise that the mechanisms involved in the actions of androgens on prostate cancer are very complex. Dr Kevin Kelly described the

KARGER

Fax + 41 61 306 12 34
E-Mail karger@karger.ch
www.karger.com

Accessible online at:
http://BioMedNet.com/karger

Prof. Don Newling
Academic Hospital, Vrije University
Polikliniek Urologie, Postbus 7057
NL–0117 MB Amsterdam (The Netherlands)
Tel. +31 204 440272, Fax +31 206 425085

phenomenon of endocrine withdrawal syndrome in patients whose cancer becomes androgen independent. The heartening news is that through studying this phenomenon we now have a clearer idea of the underlying disease processes and this will enable us to develop more rational treatment strategies.

In all walks of life the approaching millennium provokes reappraisal. This is also true for those involved in the treatment of prostate cancer. The past 50 years have seen major breakthroughs in our understanding and treatment strategies but in the new millennium we will still face major challenges in the management of this disease. These will demand ever closer co-operation between scientists and clinicians, between the laboratory and the clinic, if we are going to cure as many patients as possible who develop prostate cancer and preserve an optimal quality of life in patients with the disease who we can not cure.

European
Urology

Eur Urol 1998;34(suppl 3):3–6

J. Schalken

University Hospital Nijmegen,
The Netherlands

Molecular Diagnostics and Therapy of Prostate Cancer: New Avenues

Key Words
Prostate cancer
Molecular oncology
Biological techniques

Abstract
Co-operation and communication between clinicians and scientists is required to meet the major challenges presented by the diagnosis and therapy of prostate cancer. Molecular oncology is playing an increasing role in this field and has already been instrumental in elucidating many of the basic mechanisms underlying the development and progression of prostate cancer. By understanding these mechanisms, factors which determine whether the tumour will metastasise, such as loss of function of E-cadherin, have been identified and may help the clinician determine which therapeutic strategy is most appropriate for an individual patient. Clinicians also need more sensitive tools to help them diagnose prostate cancer and monitor its progression. The marker DD3/PCA3 shows potential in this respect. Perhaps the most fruitful area for molecular research is in the definition of new therapeutic targets useful in hormone-refractory prostate cancer. In the early stages of development are those agents which target the activation of programmed cell death, inhibition of signal transduction, inactivation of telomerase activity, and differentiation therapy. In order to accelerate the implementation of diagnostic aids and more effective therapeutic strategies for prostate cancer, clinicians must have a greater insight into the molecular mechanisms operating in their patients' disease and scientists need to understand the clinical problems involved.

Introduction

Prostate cancer and its treatment continue to present the medical community with major challenges. These are more likely to be met by translational research which requires a clear definition of clinical problems, pragmatic research plans and appropriate communication between clinicians and scientists. This will enable knowledge from research to be brought into clinical practice, and will involve looking at prostate cancer from the macroscopic viewpoint of the surgeon and the microscopic viewpoint of the cell biologist.

Molecular oncology has played an increasing role in the solution of some of the most difficult problems associated with prostate cancer therapy, and will continue to do so in the future. For example, among the most pressing clinical issues in urological oncology is the accurate determination of the biological aggressiveness of individual malignant processes which will enable clinicians to develop the best therapeutic strategy for a patient. Differential gene expression may enable more sensitive markers than prostate-specific antigen (PSA) to be identified that can be used for the follow-up of cancer progression. With this aim, over the past couple of years a number of studies

KARGER

Fax + 41 61 306 12 34
E-Mail karger@karger.ch
www.karger.com

0302–2838/98/0349–0003$15.00/0

Accessible online at:
http://BioMedNet.com/karger

Prof. Jack Schalken
Urology Research Laboratory, University Hospital
PO Box 9101
NL–6500 HB Nijmegen (The Netherlands)
Tel. +31 24361 4146, Fax +31 24354 1031, E-Mail j.schalken@mailbox.kun.nl

have been designed to identify differences in gene expression between prostate cancer cells and normal prostate epithelial cells. Molecular biological techniques are also helping with the definition and exploitation of new targets for therapy of disseminated disease.

Prostate Cancer Aggressiveness

For the accurate determination of the biological aggressiveness of a cancer in an individual patient, the molecular basis of cancer development and progression must be elucidated. When oncogenes were discovered 20 years ago a solution was thought to be imminent, but, because of the complexity of the molecular mechanisms involved, it is only recently that the process has become better understood. Four categories of genes have been identified. In the first category are genes that code for detoxifying enzymes, which are key components of the defence against carcinogenic compounds; sub-optimally performing detoxifying enzymes increase the chance of acquiring genetic mutations. The second group of genes code for DNA repair enzymes which will prevent the propagation of genetic changes within the cell population. If both classes of enzymes are not working properly, the likelihood of developing a malignant process is higher. The third group of genes is associated with the control of the cell cycle. Aberrations usually result in genetic instability. The greatest threat to the patient is usually when the malignancy metastasises. Therefore, invasion and metastasis genes are activated or inactivated. E-cadherin, which is involved in cell-to-cell interactions, is one of the proteins important for maintenance of epithelial integrity. Interference with E-cadherin-mediated interactions results in the cell becoming invasive, thus it is a critical and rate-limiting step in the progression of prostate cancer towards metastatic disease [1]. Loss of function of E-cadherin is associated with a poor prognosis [2].

Differential Gene Expression

A marker for prostate cancer which is more specific and sensitive than PSA is urgently needed for diagnosis and for monitoring progression. Recently, a number of studies have identified genes that are expressed in prostate cancer cells but not in untransformed prostate epithelial cells. Among the many identified is DD3/PCA3 [3]. Using differential display analysis, mRNA present in malignant, but not benign, prostate tissue was identified. Two major transcripts were found in a Northern blot of RNA from 45 out of 48 prostatic carcinomas; no transcripts were expressed by normal prostate or benign prostatic hyperplasia tissue. From gene database comparisons, no homology was found between the DD3 cDNA and any other genes. DD3 expression was found to be prostate specific and highly over-expressed in prostate cancer. The hope is that exploratory clinical studies will determine if this and other molecules have diagnostic, prognostic or therapeutic potential.

New Therapeutic Targets

Androgen ablation has been used as the standard therapy for prostate cancer for more than 50 years, but continuous hormonal therapy may select for hormone-refractory cells. An understanding of prostate cell biology, for example how prostate growth is controlled, is essential in order to discover new therapeutic strategies that will overcome hormone-refractory prostate cancer.

Activation of Apoptosis (Programmed Cell Death)

In tissue homeostasis there is a balance between proliferation and cell death. In cancerous growth this balance has been disrupted and needs to be redressed either by reducing proliferation or increasing the rate of apoptosis. The reduction or inhibition of cell proliferation has not been successful so far and attention has therefore turned to the induction of apoptosis. Androgen ablation leads to activation of apoptosis in prostate cells; in androgen-independent prostate cancer this no longer occurs. Fortunately, the programme for cell death is still there and can be activated pharmacologically, for instance by increasing intracellular calcium concentrations, deprivation of polyamines, or inhibiting DNA topoisomerase I. Although systemic toxicity is associated with these approaches, this may be reduced by designing a pro-drug. One such example is thapsigargin, a bound pro-drug which, in its active form, activates apoptosis by increasing intracellular calcium ion concentrations [4]. The thapsigargin pro-drug is activated by PSA and, as there are high concentrations of PSA around prostate cancer, is released at the tumour site [5]. The results of preclinical studies of thapsigargin are expected soon.

Inhibition of Signal Transduction

The prostate is a highly structured gland with hormone-modulated signalling between the compartments. The neurotrophin pathway is an important signal transduction pathway for the control of prostate homeostasis.

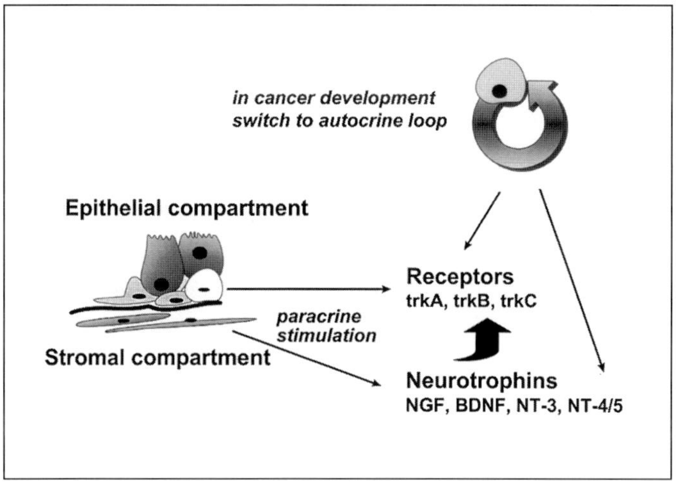

Fig. 1. The switch from paracrine to autocrine pathways in cancer development.

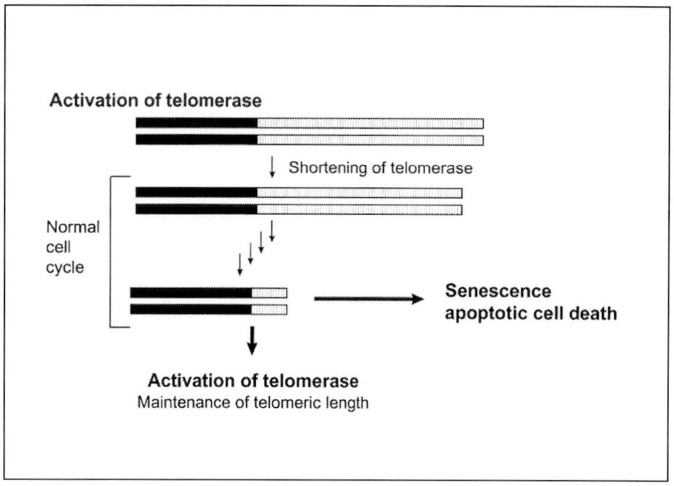

Fig. 2. The role of telomerase in the immortalised cancer cell.

By this pathway, receptors on prostate epithelial cells are intermittently activated by growth factors secreted by the stromal compartment (paracrine growth control) (fig. 1). Prostate cancer cells become independent of the stromal cells by producing both the growth factor and receptor. This autocrine loop can be broken by inhibition of signal transduction by initiation of phosphorylation of the growth factor receptor. An example of an inhibitor of growth factor receptor phosphorylation is CEP-751, a specific inhibitor of receptor tyrosine kinases [6]. In the Dunning model for rat prostate cancer, CEP-751 had an effect on androgen-dependent and androgen-independent tumours [7]. CEP-751 also had a growth inhibitory effect on human prostate cancer xenografts which is a better model for prostate cancer. Phase II clinical trials using CEP-751 are ongoing.

Inactivation of Telomerase Activity

Prostate stem cells give rise to more highly differentiated cell types in the epithelial compartment. Normal stem cells have a finite life span and cannot proliferate indefinitely; the molecular mechanism behind this is dependent on the shortening of the telomeres. At the end of the chromosome there are DNA repeats which progressively shorten with every cell division. When a critical length is reached, senescence and apoptosis are triggered. Cancer cells are rendered immortal through activation of telomerase, an enzyme which maintains the length of the telomere (fig. 2). Interference with prostate cancer cell growth by inactivation of telomerase activity may soon be tested in multinational clinical trials, e.g. by the use of deoxynucleotides [8], phosphothionate oligonucleotides [9], or hammerhead ribozymes [10].

Differentiation Therapy

Cancer progression is associated with a loss of differentiation, which can be induced by agents such as retinoic acid, 13-cis-retinoic acid, all-trans-retinoic acid, and vitamin D3. The concentrations of these compounds are significantly lower in cancer cells compared with normal cells [11]. They can be replenished exogenously but the cell may adapt by increasing metabolism [12]. In addition, their efficacy is dependent on the presence of nuclear receptors and, as in the case of high doses of retinoic acids, there may be side effects.

In another approach, the levels of naturally occurring differentiation agents are maintained by blocking their degradation. A retinoic acid metabolising blocking agent, liarozole, was tested in phase I and phase II clinical trials, but this programme was halted. Liarozole was developed as an inhibitor of cytochrome P450-dependent (adrenal) androgen synthesis, but it turned out to be an effective inhibitor of 4-hydroxylase. Nevertheless, differentiation was enhanced by up-regulation of E-cadherin production which in turn induced changes in keratin expression, and there was circumstantial evidence that retinoic acid concentrations increased [13]. An objective response was observed in patients but changes in differentiation probably did not account for all the observed clinical effects and the patient groups were not appropriate. Other retinoic acid metabolising blocking agents may enter clinical trials in the near future.

Conclusion

Over the past 5 years, new targets for the therapy of prostate cancer have been defined. Approximately 130 new drugs and gene therapies are in preclinical, phase I and phase II trials. Through an understanding of the mechanisms involved in prostate cancer, advanced molecular diagnostics can be used to tailor therapy and new therapeutic approaches can be designed. Molecular diagnostics and molecular therapy are therefore likely to become increasingly important. Effective communication between cell biologists and clinical scientists should enable new therapeutic strategies to be developed. In addition, clinicians having a greater understanding of the underlying disease processes will accelerate the implementation of research findings.

References

1 Giroldi LA, Bringuier PP, Schalken JA: Defective E-cadherin function in urological cancers: Clinical implications and molecular mechanisms. Invasion Metastasis 1994;14:71–81.

2 Umbas R, Isaacs WB, Bringuier PP, Schaafsma HE, Karthaus HF, Oosterhof GO, Debruyne FM, Schalken JA: Decreased E-cadherin expression is associated with poor prognosis in patients with prostate cancer. Cancer Res 1994;54:3929–3933.

3 Bussemakers MJG, van Bokhoven A, Debruyne FMJ: DD3: A new prostate-specific marker, strongly overexpressed in prostatic tumors. J Urol 1997;157:21 [Abs 83].

4 Lin XS, Denmeade SR, Cisek L, Isaacs JT: Mechanism and role of growth arrest in programmed (apoptotic) death of prostatic cancer cells induced by thapsigargin. Prostate 1997; 33:201–207.

5 Denmeade SR, Isaacs JT: Activation of programmed (apoptotic) cell death for the treatment of prostate cancer. Adv Pharmacol 1996; 35:281–306.

6 Camoratto AM, Jani JP, Angeles TS, Maroney AC, Sanders CY, Murakata C, Neff NT, Vaught JL, Isaacs JT, Dionne CA: CEP-751 inhibits TRK receptor tyrosine kinase activity in vitro OFF exhibits anti-tumor activity. Int J Cancer 1997;72:673–679.

7 Dionne CA, Camoratto AM, Jani JP, Emerson E, Neff N, Vaught JL, Murakata C, Djakiew D, Lamb J, Bova S, George D, Isaacs JT: Cell cycle independent death of prostate adenocarcinoma is induced by the trk tyrosine kinase inhibitor CEP-751 (KT6587). Clin Cancer Res 1998;4: 1887–1898.

8 Pai RB, Pai SB, Kukhanova M, Dutschmann GE, Guo K, Cheng YC: Telomerase from human leukemia cells: Properties and its interaction with deoxynucleoside analogues. Cancer Res 1998;58:1909–1913.

9 Mata JE, Joshi SS, Palen B, Pirruccello SJ, Jackson JD, Ellas N, Page TJ, Medlin KL, Iversen PL: A hexameric phosphorothioate oligonucleotide telomerase inhibitor arrests growth of Burkitt's lymphoma cells in vitro and in vivo. Toxicol Appl Pharmacol 1997;144: 189–197.

10 Kanazawa Y, Ohkawa K, Ueda K, Mita E, Takehara T, Sasaki Y, Kasahara A, Hayashi N: Hammerhead ribozyme-mediated inhibition of telomerase activity in extracts of human hepatocellular carcinoma cells. Biochem Biophys Res Commun 1996;225:570–576.

11 Pasquali D, Thaller C, Eichele G: Abnormal level of retinoic acid in prostate cancer tissues. J Clin Endocrinol Metab 1996;81:2186–2191.

12 Trump DL, Smith DC, Stiff D, Adedoyin A, Day R, Bahnson RR, Hofacker J, Branch RA: A phase II trial of all-trans-retinoic acid in hormone refractory prostate cancer: A clinical trial with detailed pharmacokinetic analysis. Cancer Chemother Pharmacol 1997;39:349–356.

13 De Coster R, Wouters W, Van Ginckel R, End D, Krekels M, Coene MC, Bowden C: Experimental studies with liarozole (R 75,251): An antitumoral agent which inhibits retinoic acid breakdown. J Steroid Biochem Mol Biol 1992; 43:197–201.

European
Urology

Eur Urol 1998;34(suppl 3):7–11

P. Iversen

Department of Urology, Rigshospitalet,
University of Copenhagen, Denmark

Orchidectomy and Oestrogen Therapy Revisited

Key Words
Orchidectomy
Luteinizing hormone-releasing hormone agonists
Oestrogen
Parenteral
Prostate cancer

Abstract
Over the past 20 years therapeutic options for prostate cancer have increased. Nevertheless, there may still be a role for long-established treatments such as orchidectomy and oestrogens. Orchidectomy is a simple surgical procedure, and patient survival is comparable with other treatments involving androgen ablation. However, loss of libido and sexual function is an expected outcome and hot flushes occur in about 50% of patients. Osteoporosis, loss of muscle mass, and the psychological impact associated with orchidectomy are of concern, particularly with increasing treatment periods. Nevertheless, orchidectomy is indicated when an immediate reduction of testosterone levels is required, or the patient does not comply with other treatments or objects to the cost of medical therapy. Oestrogen therapy may be superior to castration in terms of efficacy, but orally administered oestrogens are associated with gynaecomastia, loss of sexual function and unacceptable cardiovascular toxicity. Low dose oestrogens in combination with antiandrogens or antithrombotic agents may be better tolerated treatments. The route of administration is a crucial factor in the genesis of cardiovascular toxicity and parenterally administered oestrogens may not entail the same risk. Further research in this area is warranted.

Introduction

Over the past 20 years a number of new pharmacological agents for androgen deprivation have been introduced in the management of prostate cancer. Luteinizing hormone-releasing hormone (LH-RH) agonists and antiandrogens are effective, well tolerated, and widely used. In view of this, is there still a role for bilateral orchidectomy or orally administered oestrogen, the treatments of choice for many years?

In the quest for improvement in survival for patients with prostate cancer, alternative regimens such as combined androgen blockade (CAB) and intermittent androgen deprivation are being tried. The combination of surgical or pharmacological castration and an antiandrogen has been advocated based on experimental and clinical findings. However, a large US intergroup trial of almost 1,400 patients did not find the combination of orchidectomy and flutamide clinically superior to orchidectomy plus placebo [1]. This study concurs with a meta-analysis

KARGER
Fax + 41 61 306 12 34
E-Mail karger@karger.ch
www.karger.com

0302–2838/98/0349–0007$15.00/0

Accessible online at:
http://BioMedNet.com/karger

Dr. Peter Iversen
Department of Urology D 2112, Rigshospitalet
Blegdamsvej 9
DK–2100 Copenhagen (Denmark)
Tel. +45 3545 2314, Fax +45 3545 2158, E-Mail piv@rh.dk

Table 1. Indications for bilateral orchidectomy in prostate cancer patients

Immediate reduction of testosterone into castrate range is necessary, i.e. imminent spinal compression, severe pain
Poor compliance with daily medication or injections at regular intervals
Patient objects to the cost of medical therapy and opts for surgery

of 22 trials comparing CAB with castration alone (either medical or surgical) in which no statistically significant difference in survival could be found [2].

Although LH-RH agonists and antiandrogens result in greater patient acceptability, choice and timing of therapy continue to be a balance between anti-tumour efficacy and effect on quality of life. With this in mind, orchidectomy and oestrogens may still have a place in prostate cancer therapy.

Bilateral Orchidectomy

After forming part of religious and cultural practice for more than 2000 years (for example eunuchs, castrati singers, or as punishment), bilateral orchidectomy entered urological practice in the late 19th century, when it was used for treatment of prostatic enlargement with some success [3]. The use of surgical castration for control of prostate cancer began with Huggins' landmark discoveries [4].

This surgical procedure is simple and may be performed either as a total orchidectomy or by a subcapsular technique which leaves the tunica albuginea and epididymis in the scrotum. Although some people argue that testosterone-producing cells may persist following subcapsular orchidectomy, and that this operation causes slightly more complications, total and subcapsular orchidectomy may be considered similar in terms of efficacy and endocrinological consequences [5, 6]. Postoperative complications are generally few; haematoma and infections occur, but the associated morbidity in today's setting needs to be fully defined using contemporary series.

Following orchidectomy the primary source of circulating androgen is ablated and castrate levels of testosterone are reached in serum within 24 hours. The procedure is effective and is often referred to as the 'gold standard' treatment. Indeed, apart from one study finding a survival advantage for a combination of goserelin acetate and flutamide over orchidectomy [7], no other endocrine therapy has convincingly been shown to result in improved survival of patients.

Loss of libido and sexual function must be expected following orchidectomy in prostate cancer patients, although exceptions are occasionally seen. The mechanism behind bothersome hot flushes, which occur in approximately 50% of patients, has been explained by hypogonadism leading to high concentrations of adrenergic transmitter in the hypothalamus, stimulating not only LH-RH neurones but also the thermoregulatory centre [8]. The hot flushes may be effectively treated by small doses of oestrogen or steroid antiandrogens, both of which exert a negative feedback on the hypothalamic-pituitary axis, thereby reducing the outflow of adrenergic transmitter substances.

With androgen deprivation being used at earlier stages of disease, and thus for longer periods of time in younger patients, reports of osteoporosis and subsequent risk of fractures following castration have received considerable attention [9, 10]. Loss of muscle mass and lack of physical and psychological energy are also frequent, although less well described, adverse effects.

The psychological impact of surgical castration has been underestimated in the past, and several publications report that most patients prefer pharmacological castration, if given the choice [11, 12]. Nevertheless, bilateral orchidectomy continues to be the optimal endocrine manipulation in many prostate cancer patients and its indications are listed in table 1.

Is There a Difference between Orchidectomy and LH-RH Agonists?

Pharmacological castration can be achieved with LH-RH agonists. Like endogenous LH-RH, synthetic agonists stimulate the anterior pituitary to release gonadotrophins. However, continuous stimulation by potent synthetic agonists with longer half-lives than endogenous LH-RH results in down-regulation of pituitary LH-RH receptors and a paradoxical suppression of gonadotrophin secretion and sex steroid production. LH-RH agonists are polypeptides and can not be administered orally but are injected subcutaneously or intramuscularly. Depots for 1, 2 and 3 monthly use are available [13]. In men, castrate levels of testosterone in serum are generally reached within 2 weeks and are maintained for the duration of therapy [14]. In the treatment of prostate cancer, the initial stimulatory effect of LH-RH agonists occurring during the first week of treatment is associated with a risk of objective manifestations and deterioration of symptoms, referred to as the 'flare phenomenon'. Antiandrogens or oestrogens given during this initial period of LH-RH agonist therapy counteract the flare and such flare protection should be used in all patients with severe symptoms, or large tumour burdens who have a concomitant risk of spinal compression or ureteric obstruction.

Several studies have found treatment with LH-RH agonists to be comparable with surgical castration with regard to side effects and efficacy [15, 16]. However, 'head-to-head' randomized comparison between surgical castration and LH-RH agonists has only been conducted in approximately 600 patients [15, 16], and the significance of LH-RH receptors present in prostatic malignant cells, as well as the occasional 'escape' of serum testosterone to above castrate range in patients on LH-RH agonist therapy [17], is not absolutely clear. Still, LH-RH agonists represent an established and well tolerated alternative to surgical castration in endocrine manipulation of prostate cancer.

Recently, synthetic and potent LH-RH antagonists have been investigated [18]. These agents cause an immediate inhibition of the release of LH, follicle stimulating hormone, and sex steroids. Whether LH-RH antagonists have clinical potential, either alone or in combination with LH-RH agonists, awaits further research.

Table 2. Complications of oral oestrogens

Side effect	Patients, %
Impotence	97
Gynaecomastia	49–80
Peripheral oedema	16–23
Hot flushes	11–17
Nausea/gastrointestinal disturbance	4–16
Angina	2–10
Venous thrombosis	2–8
Claudication	2
Transient ischaemia	2
Phlebitis	1–7

Data from [20].

Table 3. High risk factors for cardiovascular complications during oestrogen therapy for prostate cancer

Age > 75 years
Weight > 75 kg
Pre-existing cardiovascular disease
ST-segment depression during exercise stress
Elevated serum luteinizing hormone before treatment

Oestrogens

The antigonadotrophic effect of oestrogens has been used in the treatment of prostate cancer since Huggins et al. [4] demonstrated the androgen dependency of prostate cancer. Among the many formulations of both natural and artificial oestrogens, oral diethylstilboestrol (DES) has been most frequently used, but polyoestradiol phosphate for parenteral use and ethinyl oestradiol for oral administration have also been used, particularly in Scandinavia. Both experimental and clinical evidence suggest that oestrogen therapy may be superior to castration in terms of efficacy, possibly because of a direct effect on the tumour [19–21]. Suggested effects of oestrogens are increased synthesis of sex hormone binding globulin, decreased levels of adrenal androgens presumably via a change in hepatic function, inhibition of 5-α-reductase, suppression of dedifferentiation, direct effect on Leydig cell function, and a possible cytotoxic effect [20]. However, the most important mode of action remains depression of serum testosterone. A daily oral dose of DES 3–5 mg reliably reduces serum testosterone levels to castrate range [22]. While the effect of 1 mg is less certain, in clinical studies DES 1 mg daily has never been shown to be inferior to other forms of hormonal therapy in terms of efficacy [23, 24].

Along with gynaecomastia and loss of sexual function in most treated patients, fluid retention with peripheral oedema in up to 23% of patients and deep venous thrombosis (2–8%) are also included in the known side effects associated with oestrogen therapy (table 2) [20]. However, it was unacceptable cardiovascular toxicity that severely limited the routine use of oral oestrogens. Lethal, dose-dependent cardiovascular complications have been reported in up to 16% of treated patients (DES 5 mg) compared with 11.7% in placebo-treated patients [19], and include myocardial infarction, pulmonary embolism, congestive heart failure and cerebrovascular accident. Even with DES 1 mg daily, a more modest, but still significantly increased, cardiovascular toxicity compared with orchidectomy has been reported [24]. Patients at particular risk of cardiovascular complications have been identified, as shown in table 3 [25, 26].

The route of administration of oestrogen has been demonstrated to be crucial in the genesis of cardiovascular toxicity. A high concentration of oestrogen in portal blood following oral intake exerts a 'first pass' effect on liver-derived plasma proteins, lipoproteins, and triglycerides, and causes an altered production of coagulation factors (increased factor VII and X and decreased antithrombin III) [27].

Studies have shown that *parenterally* administered oestrogens do not entail the same risk of cardiovascular complications as those administered orally [28, 29]. The value of parenterally administered oestrogen is currently being investigated in a large-scale study. This multicentre study (SPCG 5) conducted by the Scandinavian Prostatic Cancer Group, comparing polyoestradiol phosphate 240 mg intramuscularly every 4 weeks (every 2 weeks for the first 2 months) with CAB, has recently completed recruitment of more than 900 patients [30]. Survival is the final endpoint, but the double-blind protocol also includes quality of life assessment and evaluation of possible cardiovascular toxicity by blinded cardiologist observers. To date, more than 50% of patients have died and comparative analysis is ongoing.

Parallel to the increasing knowledge about the cause of cardiovascular toxicity, there is growing interest in exploring the potential extra benefits associated with oestrogen therapy for prostate cancer. Questions to be considered include how will DES 1 mg compare with castration (or CAB) in large studies, and is it possible to prevent the cardiovascular toxicity with low-dose antiplatelet agents (aspirin) or warfarin?

Low dose DES (0.1 mg daily) combined with a low dose of the steroidal antiandrogen cyproterone acetate (100 mg daily) has been used in uncontrolled series. The combination holds the promise of low toxicity and resulted in a rapid fall of serum testosterone into the castrate range [31]. Such combinations of low dose DES with steroidal or nonsteroidal antiandrogens also deserve evaluation in randomized comparative studies.

Hopefully, the studies will help to clarify the future role of oestrogens in the management of prostate cancer.

Conclusion

Bilateral orchidectomy still has a definite role to play in the treatment of patients with prostate cancer, but as more new pharmacological modalities become available concerns about quality of life issues and long-term side effects can be considered and taken into account when choosing the optimal treatment. LH-RH agonists represent an effective and valuable alternative with comparable efficacy, not requiring a major operation and having less psychological impact. However, the long-term side effects of LH-RH agonists are not expected to be different from those following surgical castration.

Oestrogen therapy is inexpensive and convenient when administered orally but has unacceptable cardiovascular toxicity. However, oestrogen therapy is associated with potential efficacy advantages in the management of prostate cancer, and studies investigating parenterally administered oestrogens, which are less likely to produce cardiovascular effects, as well as oral oestrogen combined with antithrombotic agents or antiandrogens, are warranted.

References

1 Crawford ED, Eisenberger MA, McLeod DG, Wilding G, Blumenstein BA: Comparison of bilateral orchiectomy with or without flutamide for the treatment of patients (PTS) with stage D2 adenocarcinoma of the prostate: results of NCI Intergroup Study 0105 (SWOG and ECOG). J Urol 1997;157:336[A1311].

2 Prostate Cancer Trialists' Collaborative Group: Maximum androgen blockade in advanced prostate cancer: an overview of 22 randomised trials with 3283 deaths in 5710 patients. Lancet 1995;346:265–269.

3 Glass JM, Watkin N: From mutilation to medication: the history of orchidectomy. Br J Urol 1997;80:373–378.

4 Huggins C, Hodges C: Studies on prostate cancer. I: The effect of castration, of oestrogen and of androgen injection on serum phosphatases in metastatic carcinoma of the prostate. Cancer Res 1941;1:293–297.

5 Zhang XZ, Donovan MP, Williams BT, Mohler J: Comparison of subcapsular and total orchiectomy for treatment of metastatic prostate cancer. Urology 1996;47:402–404.

6 Bergman B, Damber JE, Tomic R: Effects of total and subcapsular orchidectomy on serum concentrations of testosterone and pituitary hormones in patients with carcinoma of the prostate. Urol Int 1982;37:139–144.

7 Denis LJ, Keuppens F, Smith PH, Whelan P, de Moura JL, Newling D, Bono A, Sylvester R: Maximal androgen blockade: final analysis of EORTC phase III trial 30853. EORTC Genito-Urinary Tract Cancer Cooperative Group and the EORTC Data Center. Eur Urol 1998;33:144–151.

8 Radlmaier A, Bormacher K, Neumann F: Hot flushes: mechanism and prevention. Prog Clin Biol Res 1990;359:131–140.

9 Daniell HW: Osteoporosis after orchiectomy for prostate cancer. J Urol 1997;157:439–444.

10 Townsend MF, Sanders WH, Northway RO, Graham SD: Bone fractures associated with luteinizing hormone-releasing hormone agonists used in the treatment of prostate carcinoma. Cancer 1997;79:545–550.

11 Cassileth BR, Soloway MS, Vogelzang NJ, Schellhammer PS, Seidmon EJ, Hait HI, Kennealey GT: Patients' choice or treatment in stage D prostate cancer. Urology 1989;33 (suppl):57–62.

12 Samdal F, Vada K, Lundmo PI, Mjølnerørd OK: Orchidectomy or LHRH-analogue? Which do the patients prefer and what treatment would Norwegian urologists prefer if they had advanced cancer of the prostate? Scand J Urol Nephrol 1991;25:197–199.

13 Dijkman GA, Debruyne FMJ, Fernandez del Moral P, Plasman JWMH, Hoefakker JW, Idema JG, Sykes M: A randomised trial comparing the safety and efficacy of the Zoladex 10.8-mg depot, administered every 12 weeks, to that of the Zoladex 3.6-mg depot, administered every 4 weeks, in patients with advanced prostate cancer. Eur Urol 1995;27:43–46.
14 Conn PM, Crowley WF Jr: Gonadotrophin-releasing hormone and its analogues. N Engl J Med 1991;324:93–103.
15 Peeling WB: Phase III studies to compare goserelin (Zoladex) with orchiectomy and with diethylstilbestrol in treatment of prostatic carcinoma. Urology 1989;33(suppl):45–51.
16 Soloway MS, Smith JA, Chodak G, Scott M, Vogelzang NJ, Kennealey G, Block NL, Gau TC, Schellhammer PF: Zoladex versus orchiectomy in treatment of advanced prostate cancer: A randomised trial. Urology 1991;37:46–51.
17 Iversen P, Rose C, Stage JG, Iversen H-G, Hansen RI, Hvidt V, Mogensen P, Pedersen T, Hansen JB, and the Copenhagen Prostate Cancer Group: LHRH analogue as a depot preparation (Zoladex) in the treatment of advanced carcinoma of the prostate followed by orchiectomy as a second line therapy, a phase II study. Scand J Urol Nephrol 1989;23:177–183.
18 Pinski J, Yano T, Miller G, Schally AV: Blockade of the LH response induced by the agonist D-Trp-6-LHRH in rats by a highly potent LH-RH antagonist SB-75. Prostate 1992;20:213–224.
19 Byar DP: The Veterans Administration Cooperative Urological Research Group's studies of cancer of the prostate. Cancer 1973;32:1126–1130.
20 Cox RL, Crawford ED: Estrogens in the treatment of prostate cancer. J Urol 1995;154:1991–1998.
21 Johansson J-E, Andersson S-O, Holmberg L, Bergström R: Primary orchiectomy versus estrogen therapy in advanced prostatic cancer – a randomized study: results after 7 to 10 years of followup. J Urol 1991;145:519–523.
22 Kent JR, Bischoff AJ, Arduino LJ, Mellinger GT, Byar DP, Hill M, Kozbur X: Estrogen dosage and suppression of testosterone levels in patients with prostatic carcinoma. J Urol 1973;109:858–862.
23 Byar DP, Corle DK: Hormone therapy for prostate cancer: results of the Veterans Administration Cooperative Urological Research Group studies. Natl Cancer Inst Monogr 1988;7:165–169.
24 Robinson MRG, Smith PH, Richards B, Newling DWW, de Pauw M, Sylvester R: The final analysis of the EORTC Genito-Urinary Tract Cancer Co-operative group phase III clinical trial (protocol 30805) comparing orchidectomy, orchidectomy plus cyproterone acetate and low dose stilboestrol in the management of metastatic carcinoma of the prostate. Eur Urol 1995;28:273–283.
25 de Voogt H, Pavone-Macaluso M, Smith PH, de Pauw M, Suciu S: Lessons from phase III-trials on hormonal treatment of prostatic cancer. I: Results of EORTC-trials 30761 and 30762. Prog Clin Biol Res 1988;260:111–117.
26 Henriksson P, Edhag O, Eriksson A, Johansson SE: Patients at high risk of cardiovascular complications in oestrogen treatment of prostatic cancer. Br J Urol 1989;63:186–189.
27 von Schoultz B, Carlström K, Collste L, Eriksson A, Henriksson P, Pousette A, Stege R: Estrogen therapy and liver function: Metabolic effects of oral and parenteral administration. Prostate 1989;14:389–395.
28 Stege R, Sander S: Endocrine treatment of prostatic cancer. A renaissance for parenteral estrogen. Tidsskr Nor Laegeforen 1993;113:833–835.
29 Aro J, Haapiainen R, Rasi V, Rannikko S, Alfthan O: The effect of parenteral estrogen versus orchiectomy on blood coagulation and fibrinolysis in prostate cancer patients. Eur Urol 1990;17:161–165.
30 Hedlund PO: The Scandinavian Prostatic Cancer Group. Scand J Urol Nephrol 1997;31:5–7.
31 Goldenberg SL, Bruchovsky N: Use of cyproterone acetate in prostate cancer. Urol Clin N Am 1991;18:111–122.

European Urology

Eur Urol 1998;34(suppl 3):12–17

F.H. Schröder

Department of Urology, Erasmus University and Academic Hospital, Rotterdam, The Netherlands

Antiandrogens as Monotherapy for Prostate Cancer

Key Words
Antiandrogens
Monotherapy
Bicalutamide
Prostate cancer

Abstract
Castration or antiandrogen monotherapies remain options for prostate cancer treatment as only marginal benefits have been demonstrated with combined androgen blockade, although it may be that certain subgroups of patient may benefit. Of the nonsteroidal antiandrogens, bicalutamide 150 mg was as effective as castration in M0 patients with significant improvement in sexual interest and physical capacity, but the trial has yet to reach maturity. In M1 patients, bicalutamide 150 mg was not as effective as castration but this may be outweighed by symptomatic and quality of life benefits. Nilutamide is not recommended as monotherapy and there are little data on flutamide. The steroidal antiandrogen, cyproterone acetate, is as effective as oestrogen therapy and has a better side-effect profile, although cardiovascular and hepatic side effects are still of concern. Compared with flutamide, in a recently completed EORTC study, side effects such as gynaecomastia, diarrhoea, nausea, and liver function deterioration occurred less often, and thrombotic effects more often, in the cyproterone acetate group. No difference was seen in the preservation of sexual functioning. Quality of life issues are becoming increasingly important and thus antiandrogen monotherapy may become more widely used in the management of prostate cancer.

Introduction

Surgical or pharmacological castration will probably remain standard treatment for hormone-sensitive prostate cancer as the initial high expectations for maximal androgen blockade (MAB) or complete androgen blockade (CAB) arising from phase II and early phase III studies have not been fully realized. An increasing volume of knowledge is accumulating about the usefulness of CAB. A meta-analysis including almost all trials, published and non-published, demonstrated no significant advantage in terms of efficacy for CAB compared with castration alone [1]. Results from an update of this meta-analysis are awaited. In addition, a large, randomized, double-blind study, conducted by the South West Oncology Group, of surgical castration plus flutamide or placebo in patients with metastatic prostate cancer did not confirm the initial favourable results obtained by the same group with the similar regimen where the castration element was achieved by the administration of a luteinizing hormone-releasing hormone (LH-RH) agonist [2, 3]. Thus, although there may be only marginal benefits with CAB, attempts to identify those groups of patients that may truly benefit are still ongoing.

KARGER

Fax +41 61 306 12 34
E-Mail karger@karger.ch
www.karger.com

0302–2838/98/0349–0012$15.00/0

Accessible online at:
http://BioMedNet.com/karger

Dr. Fritz H. Schröder
Department of Urology
Erasmus University and Academic Hospital
NL–3000 DR Rotterdam (The Netherlands)
Tel. +31 10 463 3607, Fax +31 10 463 5838, E-Mail vanalphen@urol.azr.nl

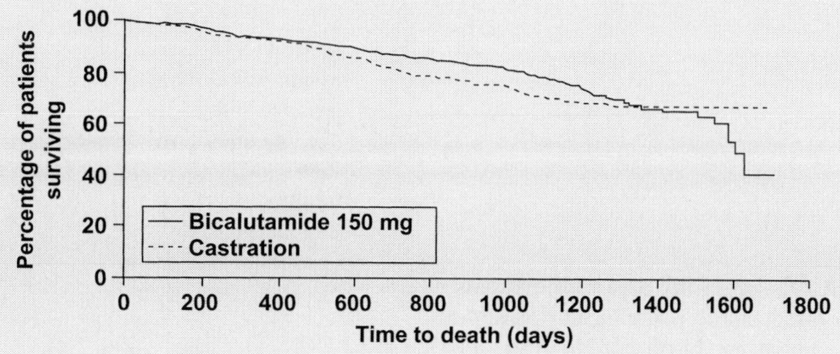

Fig. 1. Kaplan-Meier projections of survival data from patients with non-metastatic prostate cancer comparing bicalutamide 150 mg monotherapy with castration. Hazard ratio 0.93; upper one-sided 95% CI, 1.24; p = 0.67. Tails of both curves are weakly defined due to increased censoring beyond 1,200 days, i.e., they are unstable and cannot be interpreted. Adapted with permission [5].

If CAB is not necessary in every patient, is it not better to initiate endocrine treatment in a less aggressive fashion and step it up later on when progression occurs? Could endocrine treatment be applied in an intermittent fashion? Can libido and potency, at least temporarily, be preserved? Would less aggressive therapies that might be used in an adjuvant setting provide a better quality of life and decreased cost? Finally, if quality of life can really be improved for a prolonged period of time and the therapies were less effective in terms of disease-specific and overall survival, would patients be ready to exchange quality of life for life time? All of these important questions are currently being addressed and the field is now open for research into other options that have been understudied in the past.

Nonsteroidal Antiandrogens as Monotherapy

Bicalutamide

The effect of bicalutamide 50 mg, 100 mg and, more recently, 150 mg has been compared with medical or surgical castration in several studies. The dosage was escalated above 50 mg because, although an overview analysis of more than 1,000 patients showed a significant difference in favour of castration compared with bicalutamide 50 mg because of cancer-specific and overall survival, this dosage was well tolerated and showed quality of life benefits [4].

Two randomized studies of bicalutamide as monotherapy (protocols 306 and 307) included a dose-selection phase using a randomization scheme between bicalutamide 100 mg, 150 mg and castration in a ratio of 2:2:1. After the dose selection phase it was decided to continue with bicalutamide 150 mg compared with castration in a 2:1 ratio. A total of 1,453 patients were recruited to studies 306 and 307. Of these, 862 patients (320 M0, 542 M1) received bicalutamide 150 mg and 423 patients (160 M0, 263 M1) received medical or surgical castration. These studies were designed to allow a combined analysis. A protocolled interim analysis after a median follow-up of approximately 100 weeks revealed a statistically significant qualitative interaction between treatment group and stage of disease and, consequently, data from the M0 and M1 subgroups were analysed separately.

Bicalutamide 150 mg in M0 Patients

Figure 1 shows the Kaplan-Meier projections of overall survival at a median follow-up of 4 years [5]. Tails of both curves are weakly defined due to increased censoring beyond 1,200 days, i.e., they are unstable and cannot be interpreted. The hazard ratio of 0.93 favouring bicalutamide indicates that the relative risk of death was 7% lower in the bicalutamide arm relative to castration for a given period of time, although this difference was not significant. However, the 31% mortality level in this analysis is not considered to be mature.

The effects of castration and bicalutamide on parameters of quality of life are shown in figure 2. Any score of less than zero indicates a benefit for castration while scores of more than zero indicate a benefit for bicalutamide. Sexual function was also studied but the data could not be analysed because too few patients completed the relevant questions. Most of the parameters showed a positive treatment effect in favour of bicalutamide, with sexual interest and physical capacity showing statistically significant advantages (p = 0.029 and 0.046, respectively) compared with castration.

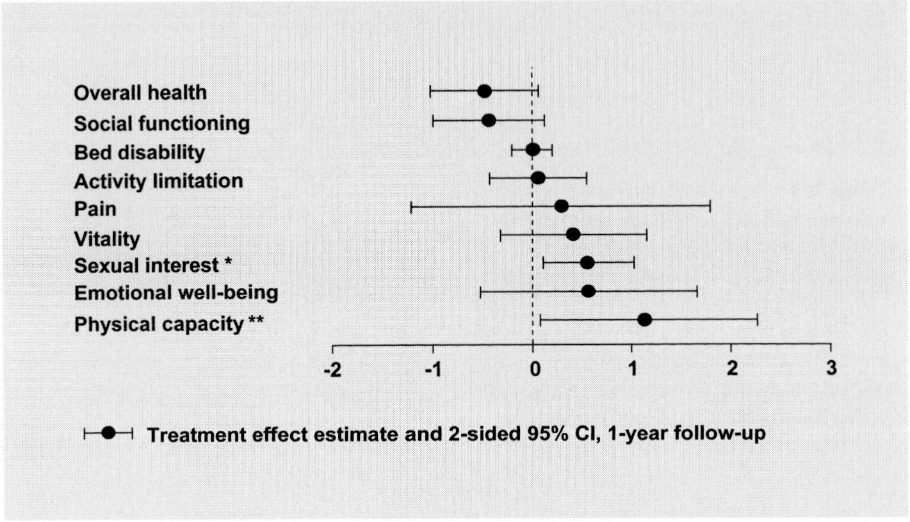

Fig. 2. Quality of life data from patients with non-metastatic, advanced prostate cancer comparing bicalutamide 150 mg monotherapy with castration. A positive treatment effect favours bicalutamide and is statistically significant where CI > 0. * p = 0.029; ** p = 0.046. Adapted with permission [5].

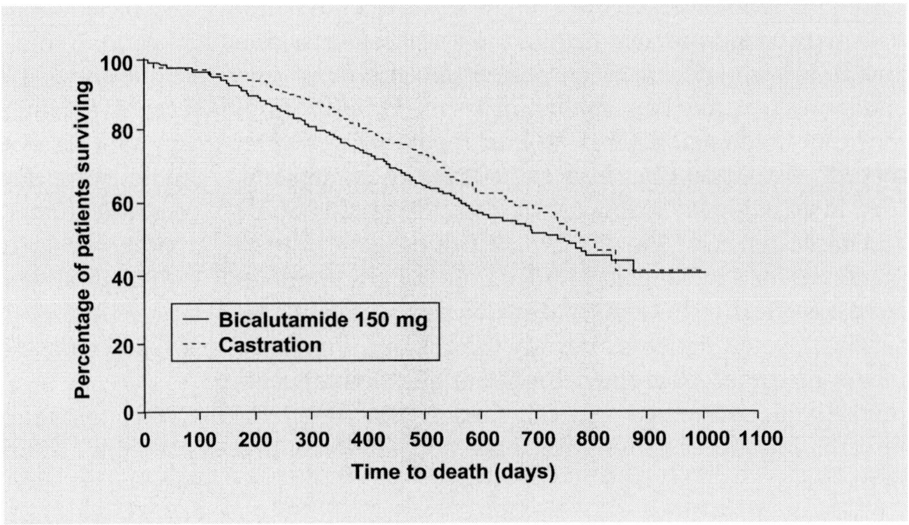

Fig. 3. Kaplan-Meier projections of survival data from patients with metastatic prostate cancer comparing bicalutamide 150 mg monotherapy with castration. Hazard ratio, 1.304; 95% CI, 1.04, 1.65; p = 0.02. Adapted with permission [6].

Bicalutamide 150 mg in M1 Patients

In the analysis of data from M1 patients, with a median follow-up of 100 weeks, castration was superior to bicalutamide 150 mg with respect to time to death with a hazard ratio of 1.304. Although this difference was statistically significant (fig. 3), the numerical difference in median survival was only 42 days (6 weeks) [6]. Again, most of the parameters, including sexual function, showed a positive treatment effect in favour of bicalutamide (fig. 4), with sexual interest and physical capacity showing statistically significant advantages (p = 0.041 and p = 0.032, respectively) compared with castration. In addition, in symptomatic patients, a significant palliative benefit was found. The 6-week difference in estimated time to death may be acceptable given the improvements in quality of life and symptomatic benefit. Therefore, bicalutamide certainly remains a treatment option when castration is not acceptable. However, the side-effect profile of bicalutamide has to be considered; the most frequent side effects are breast tenderness and gynaecomastia which occurs to a similar extent with flutamide monotherapy, in about 40% of patients [6, 7] although only 6 patients (0.75%) withdrew as a result. A form of prevention of gynaecomastia that has the potential for fewer side effects than preventive radiotherapy to the nipples is needed.

Nilutamide and Flutamide

Nilutamide is not recommended for monotherapy by the manufacturer and only minimal data are available. Flutamide has been studied in about 700 patients in a ran-

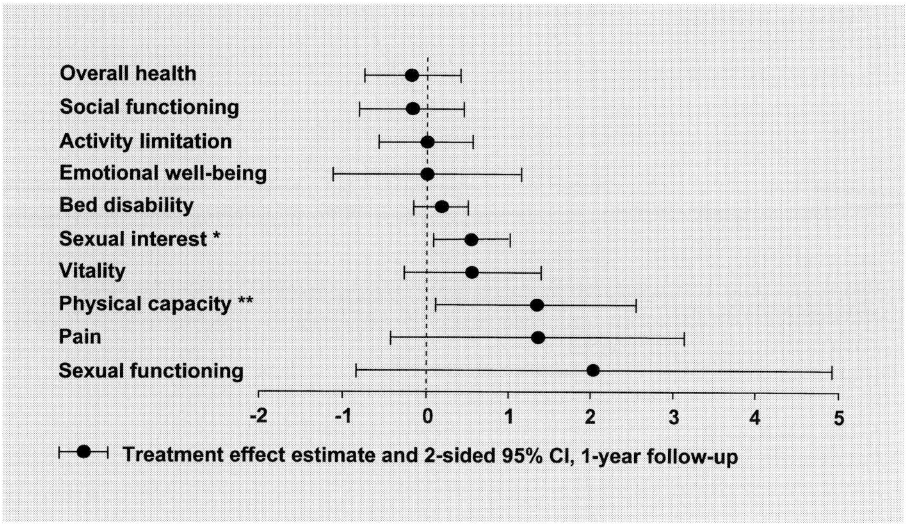

Fig. 4. Quality of life data from patients with metastatic prostate cancer comparing bicalutamide 150 mg monotherapy with castration. A positive treatment effect favours bicalutamide and is statistically significant where CI > 0. * p = 0.041; ** p = 0.032. Adapted with permission [6].

domized fashion, usually in comparison with oestrogens [8–14]. A summary of phase III studies with flutamide monotherapy is shown in table 1 [15]. In most of these relatively small studies, there were no significant differences with respect to response and survival rates. However, a large and conclusive study of flutamide versus castration or another standard form of treatment has not yet been done and the question of whether flutamide monotherapy can be considered standard treatment of prostate cancer can not be answered from the information currently available.

Table 1. Phase III studies comparing flutamide with oestrogen or castration

Comparator	Comparator/ flutamide, n	Response rate, %	Survival (months)	Ref.
DES 1 mg	7/7	NS	NS	8
DES 1 mg	44/81	NS	NS	9
DES 3 mg	20/20	NS	NS	10
DES 3 mg	40/44	F = DES	DES > F	11
EP 280 mg × 2	12/14	F > EP	NS	12
Orchidectomy	50/54	NS	NS	13
CAB	146/170	NS	NS	14

CAB, combined androgen blockade; DES, diethylstilboestrol; EP, estramustine phosphate; F, flutamide.

Adapted with permission [15].

Steroidal Antiandrogens as Monotherapy

Cyproterone acetate (CPA) is a potent steroidal antiandrogen and has gestagenic properties leading to suppression of luteinizing hormone and testosterone production. Theoretically, CPA has to cope with lower concentrations of androgens at the target cell than nonsteroidal antiandrogens. However, this theoretical advantage has not yet translated into a clinical benefit compared with therapies such as the use of oestrogens. In contrast to nonsteroidal antiandrogens and oestrogens, gynaecomastia is rarely seen with CPA. However, there are concerns about cardiovascular and hepatic side effects.

CPA was established as a therapy for prostate cancer by a number of early studies, including the European Organization for Research and Treatment of Cancer (EORTC) protocol 30761 which compared CPA 250 mg with diethylstilboestrol (DES) 3 mg [16]. No differences between M0 and M1 patients were shown with respect to cancer progression and overall survival, and the side-effect profile compared favourably with that of DES 3 mg [17]. However, in the absence of a group treated by castration, no conclusive evidence on the cardiovascular side-effect profile of CPA could be produced. Hepatic side effects were not observed in protocol 30761.

Recently, initial results of another comparative study of CPA have become available. Protocol 30892 of EORTC Genitourinary Group compared flutamide monotherapy with CPA monotherapy in untreated metastatic prostate cancer patients with favourable prognostic factors and no active cardiovascular disease. A total of 308 patients were recruited between 1990 and 1996, and the study was closed on 1 April 1996. While results of

Table 2. Patients experiencing side effects of flutamide and cyproterone acetate (CPA)*

	No. patients (%)		p
	flutamide (n = 130)	CPA (n = 134)	
Painful gynaecomastia	59 (45.4)	10 (7.5)	0.001
Diarrhoea	30 (23.1)	13 (9.7)	<0.001
Nausea	25 (19.2)	8 (6.0)	0.002
Deterioration in liver function	13 (10.0)	6 (4.5)	0.045
Thrombosis, embolus	0	6 (4. 5)	0.011

* Only those side effects that showed a significant difference between the treatment groups are included.
Adapted with permission [18].

effectiveness are still pending, side effects and sexual function have been evaluated [18]. The differences in side effects between flutamide and CPA are shown in table 2. Gynaecomastia, diarrhoea, nausea and liver function deterioration occurred more frequently with flutamide; thrombotic events were seen more frequently with CPA. However, the incidence of myocardial infarction and cerebrovascular accident did not differ between the groups. Moreover, hot flushes, for which CPA is supposed to be protective, were not a problem in either group. One of the reasons for doing the study was the hope that sexual function might be preserved in the flutamide group and that flutamide monotherapy would therefore produce a significant improvement in terms of quality of life. Unfortunately, this hope was not realized. While 33% of patients at entry claimed to have spontaneous nocturnal erections, only 25% were sexually active. This sexual activity was lost in both treatment groups within 2–3 years in 80% of patients. In line with earlier findings [19], only about 20% of sexually active men remained so after treatment with CPA or flutamide for more than 2 years. However, loss of sexual function with CPA or flutamide is a slow process and perhaps the use of intermittent treatment schemes may lead to continuous preservation of sexual function.

The Future of Endocrine Therapy

The field of endocrine treatment of prostate cancer has now reopened to considerations which include quality of life, cost, the possibility of 'step up treatment', intermittent therapy and other options which, over the past 15 years, have been understudied because of the concentration of clinical research on CAB. Also, earlier diagnosis of prostate cancer over recent years has resulted in fewer patients presenting with M1 disease. The proportion of locally confined disease, an indication for adjuvant treatment after potentially curative forms of management such as radiotherapy or radical prostatectomy, is significantly increasing. Endocrine treatment in this type of patient will require much longer treatment periods, and minimization of side effects at all levels is desirable with quality of life issues becoming more important in the future. Nonsteroidal antiandrogen monotherapy may offer such an option (as shown by the latest results with bicalutamide). If advantages in quality of life, particularly in relation to libido and potency, continue to be shown it is likely that patients may prefer nonsteroidal antiandrogen monotherapy even if, as in the case of patients with M1 disease, there is a slight shortening of their life span.

Standard treatments should be compared with 'step up' therapy, i.e., from minimally invasive forms of treatment such as 5-α-reductase inhibitors, escalating to more invasive forms of endocrine treatment. Adjuvant endocrine treatment of prostate cancer has been grossly understudied. Recent studies show that neoadjuvant endocrine treatment before radiotherapy and adjuvant treatment after radiotherapy have a significant effect on prostate cancer mortality and overall survival [20, 21]. These data need to be confirmed and followed up by studies to elucidate the necessary time schedule as well as efficacy at different stages of the disease. Thus, research into the optimization of endocrine management of prostate cancer is wide open.

Conclusion

New ways of managing prostate cancer that improve quality of life, as well as increasing the life span of the patient, are being investigated. Bicalutamide has tolerability and quality of life benefits compared with other treatments, and as more information becomes available nonsteroidal antiandrogen monotherapy may play an increasing role in the treatment of prostate cancer.

Acknowledgements

I should like to thank the members of the EORTC Genitourinary Group and the statistician of the EORTC Genitourinary Group, Mrs Laurence Collette, Brussels, for their input into this paper.

References

1 Prostate Cancer Trialists' Collaborative Group: Maximum androgen blockade in advanced prostate cancer: an overview of 22 randomised trials with 3283 deaths in 5710 patients. Lancet 1995;346:265–269.

2 Eisenberger M, Crawford ED, McLeod D, Loehrer P, Wilding G, Blumenstein B: A comparison of bilateral orchiectomy (orch) with or without flutamide in stage D2 prostate cancer (PC) (NCI INT-0105 SWOG/ECOG). 33rd Annual Meeting of the American Society of Clinical Oncology (ASCO) 1997:A1311.

3 Crawford ED, Eisenberger MA, McLeod DG, Spaulding JT, Benson R, Dorr FA, Blumenstein BA, Davis MA, Goodman PJ: A controlled trial of leuprolide with and without flutamide in prostatic carcinoma. N Engl J Med 1989;321:419–424.

4 Bales GT, Chodak GW: A controlled trial of bicalutamide versus castration in patients with advanced prostate cancer. Urology 1996; 47(suppl 1A):38–43.

5 Iversen P, Tyrrell CJ, Kaisary AV, Anderson JB, Baert L, Tammela T, Chamberlain M, Carroll K, Blackledge GRP: 'Casodex' (bicalutamide) 150 mg monotherapy compared with castration in patients with previously untreated non-metastatic prostate cancer: results from two multicentre randomized trials at median follow-up of 4 years. Urology 1998;51:389–396.

6 Tyrrell CJ, Kaisary AV, Iversen P, Anderson JB, Baert L, Tammela T, Chamberlain M, Webster A, Blackledge G: A randomised comparison of Casodex (bicalutamide) 150 mg monotherapy versus castration in the treatment of metastatic and locally advanced prostate cancer. Eur Urol 1998; in press.

7 Tyrrell CJ: Tolerability and quality of life aspects with the antiandrogen Casodex (ICI 176, 334) as monotherapy for prostate cancer. International Casodex investigators. Eur Urol 1994; 26(suppl 1):15–19.

8 Jacobo E, Schmidt JD, Weinstein SH, Flocks RH: Comparison of flutamide (SCH-13521) and diethylstilbestrol in untreated advanced prostatic cancer. Urology 1976;8:231–233.

9 Neri RO, Kassem NY: Biological and clinical properties of antiandrogens. Prog Cancer Res Ther 1984;31:507–518.

10 Lund F, Rasmussen F: Flutamide versus stilboestrol in the management of advanced prostatic cancer: A controlled prospective study. Br J Urol 1988;61:140–142.

11 Chang A, Yeap B, Davis T, Blum R, Hahn R, Khanna O, Fisher H, Rosenthal J, Witte R, Schinella R, Trump D: Double blind randomized study of primary hormonal treatment of stage D2 prostate carcinoma: flutamide versus diethylstilbestrol. J Clin Oncol 1996;14:2250–2257.

12 Johansson JE, Andersson SO, Beckman KW, Lingardh G, Zador G: Clinical evaluation of flutamide and estramustine as initial treatment of metastatic carcinoma of prostate. Urology 1987;29:55–59.

13 Boccon-Gibod L, Fournier G, Bottet P, Maréchal JM, Guiter J, Rischmann P, Hubert J, Soret JY, Mangin P, Mallo C, Fraysse CE: Flutamide versus orchidectomy in patients with metastatic prostate carcinoma. Eur Urol 1997;32: 391–395.

14 Pavone-Macaluso M: Flutamide monotherapy versus combined androgen blockade in advanced prostate cancer. Interim report of an Italian multicenter, randomised study. 23rd Congress of the Société Internationale d'Urologie (SIU) 1994, A354.

15 Boccon-Gibod L: Are non-steroidal antiandrogens appropriate as monotherapy in advanced prostate cancer? Eur Urol 1998;33: 159–164.

16 Pavone-Macaluso M, de Voogt HJ, Viggiano G, Barasolo E, Lardennois B, de Pauw M, Sylvester R: Comparison of diethylstilbestrol, cyproterone acetate and medroxyprogesterone acetate in the treatment of advance prostatic cancer: final analysis of a randomized phase III trial of the European Organization for Research on Treatment of Cancer Urological Group. J Urol 1986;136:624–631.

17 De Voogt HJ, Smith PhH, Pavone-Macaluso M, de Pauw M, Suciu S, on behalf of the EORTC-GU Group: Cardiovascular side effects of diethylstilbestrol, cyproterone acetate, medroxyprogesterone acetate and estramustine phosphate used for the treatment of advanced prostatic cancer: Results from European Organization for Research on Treatment of Cancer Trials 30761 and 30762. J Urol 1986;135:303–307.

18 Schröder FH, Whelan P, Kurth R, Sylvester R, de Pauw M and members of the EORTC Genitourinary Group: Antiandrogens as monotherapy for metastatic prostate cancer: A preliminary report on EORTC protocol 30892; in Schröder FH (ed): Recent advances in prostate cancer. London, Parthenon, 1997, pp 141–146.

19 Ellis WJ, Grayhack JT: Sexual function in aging males after orchiectomy and estrogen therapy. J Urol 1963;89:895–899.

20 Pollack A, Zagars GK: Androgen ablation in addition to radiation therapy for prostate cancer: Is there a true benefit? Semin Radiat Oncol 1998;8:95–106.

21 Bolla M, Gonzalez D, Warde P, Dubois JB, Mirimanoff R-O, Storme G, Bernier J, Kuten A, Sternberg C, Gil T, Collette L, Pierart M: Improved survival in patients with locally advanced prostate cancer treated with radiotherapy and goserelin. N Engl J Med 1997;337:295–300.

European Urology

Eur Urol 1998;34(suppl 3):18–23

W.K. Kelly

Genitourinary Oncology Service,
Department of Medicine,
Memorial Sloan-Kettering Cancer Center,
New York, N.Y., USA

Endocrine Withdrawal Syndrome and Its Relevance to the Management of Hormone Refractory Prostate Cancer

Key Words
Endocrine withdrawal syndrome
Flutamide
Bicalutamide
Androgen independent
Prostate cancer

Abstract
Therapeutic options for patients with metastatic prostate cancer relapsing from primary hormonal therapy are limited. On the selective discontinuation of flutamide in patients that have relapsed on combined androgen ablation, a third of the patients will show a significant clinical benefit for 4–6 months. A multivariate model has identified prolonged exposure to combined androgen blockade, high baseline alkaline phosphatase and prolonged flutamide exposure as prognostic factors for patients that have a significant prostate-specific antigen (PSA) decline after the withdrawal of flutamide. This phenomenon has also been described with bicalutamide and other antiandrogens, and thus has been more appropriately renamed the endocrine withdrawal syndrome. The molecular basis for this endocrine withdrawal syndrome is not completely understood but data suggest that mutations in the androgen receptor may be responsible for the paradoxical effect observed. Recognition of this syndrome has introduced a non-toxic therapy for advanced prostate cancer patients and has had a dramatic impact on the interpretation and design of clinical trials in patients with 'hormone refractory disease'.

Introduction

Patients with metastatic prostate cancer receiving androgen suppression usually experience a rise in prostate-specific antigen (PSA) concentration in a median of 2 years after initiation of therapy [1]. Once patients relapse, second-line endocrine therapy may produce a brief clinical response in 20–40% of patients, but all progress to become androgen independent and hormone insensitive (hormone refractory). The median survival for these patients is less than 1 year. Additional therapy for the hormone-resistant tumours is limited and consists of palliative therapy with chemotherapy or radiotherapy. Thus, new treatment strategies are needed for this disease.

In 1989, Wilding et al. [2] showed that the active metabolite of flutamide, hydroxyflutamide, could stimulate the growth of LNCaP cell line. Four years later, the clinical significance of this finding was elucidated when four patients with progressive metastatic prostate cancer on combined androgen blockade were shown to have an objective, biochemical and subjective improvement on

KARGER

Fax + 41 61 306 12 34
E-Mail karger@karger.ch
www.karger.com

0302–2838/0349–0018$15.00/0

Accessible online at:
http://BioMedNet.com/karger

Dr. Wm. Kevin Kelly
Genitourinary Oncology Service, Department of Medicine
Memorial Sloan-Kettering Cancer Center, 1275 York Avenue
New York, NY 10021 (USA)
Tel. +1 212 639 7992, Fax +1 212 794 5813, E-Mail kellyw@mskcc.org

selective discontinuation of flutamide [3]. This finding was confirmed by Dupont et al. [4], who reported 32 (80%) out of 40 patients on total androgen blockade had a greater than 50% decline in PSA concentration from baseline when flutamide was discontinued.

Elucidation of the 'Flutamide Withdrawal Syndrome'

This phenomenon was further characterized in 36 patients on combined androgen blockade (CAB) with either orchidectomy or luteinizing hormone-releasing hormone (LH-RH) agonist plus flutamide who were treated prospectively with the withdrawal of flutamide and observed for a response. Ten (29%) out of 35 patients that presented with a rising prostate-specific antigen (PSA) concentration had a significant decline in the marker after the discontinuation of flutamide [5]. Seven of these patients had a greater than 80% decline in PSA concentration and three achieved a 50% decline from the baseline value [5]. While the median duration of response was brief (median 4 to 6 months), all responders had dramatic improvement in their cancer-related symptoms. This series was expanded to 57 consecutive patients and 16 (28%) out of 57 had a greater than 50% decline in PSA for a median of 5 months [6].

Since the original description of 'flutamide withdrawal syndrome', multiple reports have been published evaluating the frequency of this effect. Overall, 96 (34.7%) out of 276 cases that have been reported showed a 50% or greater decline in PSA concentration from baseline with duration of responses ranging from 3.3 to 14.5 months (median 4 months) [7]. Some investigators have enhanced the clinical effect of flutamide withdrawal by simultaneously adding a second-line hormonal therapy. Sartor et al. [8] found that 48% of the patients had a 50% or more decline in the baseline PSA for a median of 8 months when aminoglutethimide and hydrocortisone were added.

Prognostic factors that identified patients with a high probability of responding to the withdrawal of flutamide were evaluated in 57 patients at Memorial Sloan-Kettering Cancer Center [6]. A multivariate model identified initial therapy with CAB, higher baseline alkaline phosphatase levels, and longer exposure to flutamide as the most significant variables associated with patients having a 50% decline in baseline PSA at 12 weeks [6]. Most series with flutamide withdrawal identified the duration of flutamide exposure to be an important predictor of outcome. Combined results of these studies demonstrated that the median time of exposure to flutamide was longer in responders (>25 months) compared with non-responders (14 months) [7]. Others have suggested that low androgen levels were predictive. A study by Herrada et al. [9] showed that patients with response after flutamide withdrawal had lower concentrations of dehydroepiandrosterone, an intermediary in the biosynthesis of testosterone, compared with non-responders.

While this phenomenon was first described with flutamide, others have reported similar withdrawal effects with bicalutamide, megestrol acetate, diethylstilboestrol, chlormadinone acetate, and cis-retinoic acid (table 1) [10–17]. The proportion of patients involved and the durability of the responses to these agents are similar to flutamide except patients withdrawn from bicalutamide may take longer to respond due to the long half-life of bicalutamide [12]. Therefore, patients withdrawn from bicalutamide may need a longer observation period to see if a withdrawal response will occur. Flutamide withdrawal syndrome has been more appropriately renamed the 'endocrine withdrawal syndrome'.

Aetiology of the Endocrine Withdrawal Syndrome

The molecular basis for the endocrine withdrawal syndrome is not completely understood. However, observations of the increased growth of the LNCaP cell line in response to the active metabolite of flutamide, hydroxyflutamide [2], and subsequent discovery of a point mutation at codon 877 in the cell line prompted speculation that mutations in the androgen receptor are involved [18]. The implications of this hypothesis for endocrine withdrawal syndrome are depicted in figure 1 [19]. In a normal situation testosterone enters the prostate cell and is converted to dihydrotestosterone, which then binds to the androgen receptor, and transcription is activated. When flutamide is added it is converted to hydroxyflutamide within the cell, binds to the androgen receptor and blocks transcription. In a cell with a mutated androgen receptor, hydroxyflutamide binds to the receptor but increases activation: transcription is increased, and subsequently translation and promotion of cell proliferation occurs.

The reported frequency of androgen receptor mutations is variable, ranging from 0 to 44% (table 2) [20–30]. This may be due to heterogeneity of the specimens used for analysis (primary versus metastatic lesions), variability of the hormonal status of the tumour (androgen dependent versus androgen independent), or different

Table 1. Reports of the endocrine withdrawal syndrome

Reference	Endocrine agent	Adjuvant treatment	>50% decline in PSA	Median exposure (months)	Time to response (weeks)	Duration of response (months)
6	Flutamide	None	16/57 (28%)	16	5.6	4
4	Flutamide	Aminoglutethimide plus hydrocortisone	32/40 (80%)	57	NA	14.5
9	Flutamide	None	11/39 (28%)	19	<6	3.3
8	Flutamide	Aminoglutethimide plus hydrocortisone	14/29 (48%)	27	<4	8
10	Flutamide	None	7/21 (33%)	28	<6	3.7
11	Flutamide	None	12/82 (15%)	21.5	NA	3.5
12	Flutamide	None	4/8 (50%)	NA	<4	NA
12	Bicalutamide	None	4/14 (29%)	NA	>7	NA
13	Bicalutamide	None	1/3 (33%)	26	<4	6
14	Megestrol	None	1/1	36	<4	5+
15	Diethylstilboestrol	None	1/1	96	NA	36+
16	Chlormadinone acetate	None	2/2	16.5	<5	NA
17	13-cis-retinoic acid	Interferon	1/1	11	<6	5+

NA, not available; PSA, prostate-specific antigen.

Table 2. Mutations and alterations in the androgen receptor

Ref.	No. patients	Mutation	Comment
20	0/5	NA	
20	1/46	$CAG_{24\rightarrow18}$	Decrease in CAG repeat in patient with response to flutamide withdrawal
21	1/26	Codon 730	Two patients with refractory disease had no mutations; exons 5–8 evaluated
22	11/25	Codons 265, 572, 268, 54, 889, 57, 111, 64, 828, 526, 670, 179, 780, 668, 789, 794	Mutations found in exons 1, 2, 4, 6, 7, 8; one tumour with increased number of CAG repeats
23	0/10	NA	
24	1/8	Codons 701, 877	
25	2/10	Codons 340, 798	
26	0/9, 0/18	NA	
27	6/24	Codon 877	
28	5/10	Codons 877, 874, 902, 721, 647*, 724*, 880*, 896*	*One patient with multiple mutations
29	8/30	Codons 760, 794, 828, 841, 889	
20	1/7	Codon 715	Transactivation with dehydroepiandrosterone, androstenedione, and progesterone
30	7/23	Amplification of androgen receptor	No mutations at codon 877; no androgen receptor amplification in untreated primary specimens

NA, not applicable.

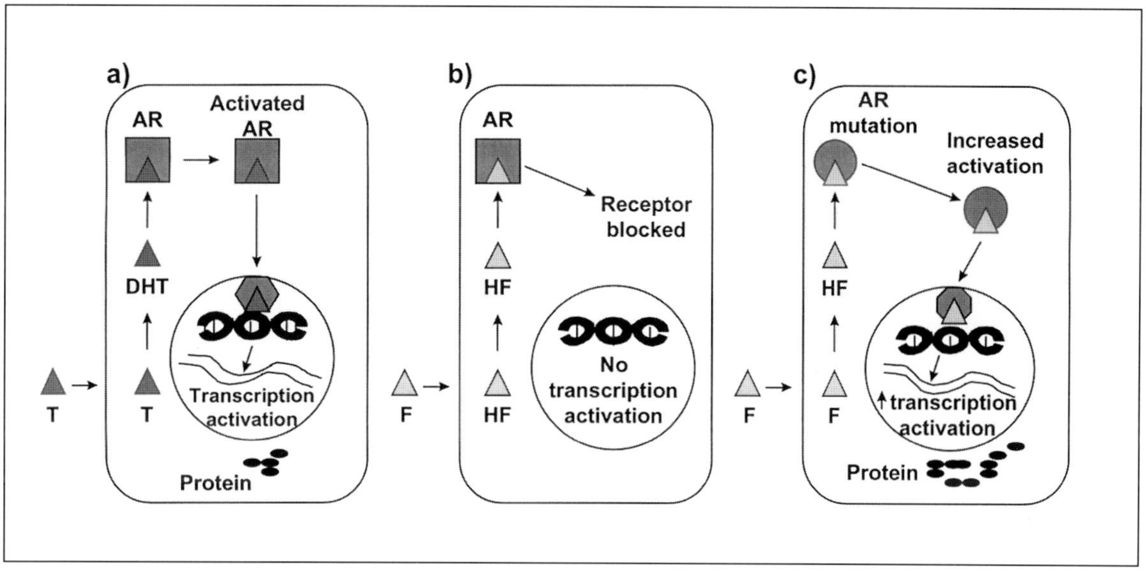

Fig. 1. Proposed molecular basis for endocrine withdrawal syndrome: **a,b** a prostate cancer cell with a normal androgen receptor; **c** a prostate cancer cell with a mutated androgen receptor. AR, androgen receptor; DHT, dihydrotestosterone; F, flutamide; HF, hydroxyflutamide; T, testosterone. Adapted with permission [19].

regions of the androgen receptor being analysed (ligand binding domain versus the complete androgen receptor). It has also been suggested that withdrawal responses may be due to clones of tumour cells that are hypersensitive to low levels of androgens and are stimulated by residual androgens or other androgen-like factors [6].

Impact of Previous Endocrine Treatment on Response

The data derived from the clinical observations of endocrine withdrawal suggest that these tumours remain hormone sensitive and additional endocrine manipulations may provide additional benefit. Several trials have evaluated the impact of second-line hormone therapy with bicalutamide in patients relapsing from primary hormonal therapy. One trial treated 51 patients with high-dose bicalutamide, 200 mg daily, and evaluated their response based on the patients' previous hormonal therapy [31]. The authors found that most of the responses to the bicalutamide were in patients that had previously been exposed to flutamide, irrespective of whether the patient had flutamide withdrawal syndrome. Patients that had monotherapy with orchidectomy or LH-RH agonist only, without flutamide, and patients treated with more than two prior hormonal manipulations had a poor response to the addition of high-dose bicalutamide [31]. This suggests that flutamide may select clones of cells that may be sensitive to bicalutamide. Joyce et al. [32] performed a similar study using bicalutamide, 150 mg daily, in patients relapsing from primary hormonal therapy. In addition to evaluating the changes in biochemical markers and measurable disease, bone marrow biopsies were performed in tumour-bearing bone for the evaluation of the androgen receptor. This study also showed that most responders had previously been exposed to flutamide. Of the patients who had previously had flutamide therapy, 43% had a significant decline in PSA concentration compared with 6% of the patients who had not been exposed to flutamide [32]. Evaluation of the androgen receptors showed mutations at codon 877 only in samples taken from patients who had received flutamide, suggesting that flutamide had a specific selective effect [32].

Conclusion

Endocrine withdrawal is a non-toxic therapeutic manoeuvre which benefits a significant number of patients with androgen-independent prostate cancer who have had a prolonged exposure to CAB. Aetiology of the withdrawal syndrome is thought to involve mutations in the androgen receptor; however, more prospective studies are needed to confirm this relationship. More importantly, the identification of the endocrine withdrawal syndrome has redefined androgen-independent disease. In the past, once patients relapsed from primary androgen ablation, the tumours were considered refractory to further endocrine manipulations. However, a proportion of these patients continue to show clinical benefit to the withdrawal of antiandrogens or the addition of secondary hormonal therapies. These tumours should be considered androgen independent and hormone sensitive. Once progression is documented after secondary endocrine manipulations these tumours are androgen independent and hormone insensitive or truly 'hormone refractory'. This classification of hormonal status has significant implications in clinical trial designs because many treatments for refractory disease include endocrine therapies as part of the therapeutic regimen [33]. The relative contribution of the endocrine component of the regimen can confound the results. Future clinical trials need to control for the effects of endocrine withdrawal, consider the hormonal status of the patient and capitalize on the ability of prior therapies to influence the biology and sensitivity of the relapsing tumour.

References

1 Newling DW, Dennis L, Vermeylen K: Orchiectomy versus goserelin and flutamide in the treatment of newly diagnosed metastatic prostate cancer. Cancer Suppl 1993;72:3793–3798.

2 Wilding G, Chen M, Gelmann EP: Aberrant response in vitro of hormone-responsive prostate cancer cells to antiandrogens. Prostate 1989;14:103–114.

3 Kelly WK, Scher HI: Prostate specific antigen decline after antiandrogen withdrawal. J Urol 1993;149:607–609.

4 Dupont A, Gomez J, Cusan L, Koutsilieris M, Labrie F: Response to flutamide withdrawal in advanced prostate cancer in progression under combination therapy. J Urol 1993;150:908–913.

5 Scher HI, Kelly WK: The flutamide withdrawal syndrome: its impact on clinical trials in hormone-refractory prostatic cancer. J Clin Oncol 1993;11:1566–1572.

6 Scher HI, Zhang Z, Cohen L, Kelly WK: Hormonally relapsed prostatic cancer: lessons from the flutamide withdrawal syndrome. Adv Urol 1995;8:61–95.

7 Kelly WK, Slovin SF, Scher HI: Steroid hormone withdrawal syndrome; in Oesterling JE (ed): Prostate Specific Antigen: The Best Prostatic Tumor Marker. Philadelphia, Saunders, 1997, pp 421–431.

8 Sartor O, Cooper M, Weinberger M, Headlee D, Tompkins A, Steinberg S, Figgs WD, Linehan WM, Myers CE: Surprising activity of flutamide withdrawal, when combined with aminoglutethimide, in treatment of 'hormone-refractory' prostate cancer. J Natl Cancer Inst 1994;86:222–227.

9 Herrada J, Dieringer P, Logothetis CJ: Characterization of patients with androgen-independent prostatic carcinoma whose serum prostate specific antigen decreased following flutamide withdrawal. J Urol 1996;155:620–623.

10 Figg WD, Sartor O, Cooper MR, Thibault A, Bergan RC, Dawson N, Reed E, Myers CE: Prostate specific antigen decline following the discontinuation of flutamide in patients with stage D2 prostate cancer. Am J Med 1995;98:412–414.

11 Small EJ, Srinivas S: The antiandrogen withdrawal syndrome: experience in a large cohort of unselected patients with advanced prostate cancer. Cancer 1995;76:1428–1434.

12 Small EJ, Schellhammer P, Venner G, Haas P, Nieh D, Seabaugh AL, Patterson E, Klein E, Wajsman Z, Furr B, Chen Y, Kennealey GT, Kolvenbag G: A double-blind assessment of antiandrogen withdrawal from casodex (C) or eulexin (E) therapy while continuing luteinizing hormone releasing hormone analogue (LHRH-a) therapy for patients with stage d2 prostate cancer. J Urol 1997;157:1731–1735.

13 Nieh PT: Withdrawal phenomenon with the antiandrogen casodex. J Urol 1995;153:1070–1073.

14 Dawson NA, McLeod DG: Dramatic prostate specific antigen decrease in response to discontinuation of megestrol acetate in advanced prostate cancer: expansion of the antiandrogen withdrawal syndrome. J Urol 1995;153:1946–1947.

15 Bissada NK, Kaczmarek AT: Complete remission of hormone refractory adenocarcinoma of the prostate in response to withdrawal of diethylstilbesterol. J Urol 1995;153:1944–1945.

16 Akakura K, Akimoto S, Ohki T, Shimazaki J: Antiandrogen withdrawal syndrome in prostate cancer after treatment with steroidal antiandrogen chlormadinone acetate. Urology 1998; in press.

17 Kelly WK, Curley T, Liebertz C, Kim B, Scher H: Phase II trial of 13-cis retinoic acid and interferon-alpha 2a in patients with adenocarcinoma of the prostate (abstract). Proc Am Soc Clin Oncol 1996;15:254.

18 Middleman MN, Lush RM, Figg WD: The mutated androgen receptor and its implications for the treatment of metastatic carcinoma of the prostate. Pharmacotherapy 1996;16:376–381.

19 Moul JW, Srivastava S, McLeod DG: Molecular implications of the antiandrogen withdrawal syndrome. Semin Urol 1995;13:157–163.

20 Culig Z, Klocker H, Eberle J, Kaspar F, Hobisch A, Cronauer M, Bartsch G: DNA sequence of the androgen receptor in prostatic tumor cell lines and tissue specimens assessed by means of the polymerase chain reaction. Prostate 1993;22:11–22.

21 Schoenberg MP, Hakimi JM, Wang S, Bova GS, Epstein JI, Fischbeck KH, Isaacs WB, Walsh PC, Barrack ER: Microsatellite mutation (CAG24→18) in the androgen receptor gene in human prostate cancer. Biochem Biophys Res Commun 1994;198:74–80.

22 Tilley WD, Buchanan G, Hickey TE, Bentel JM: Mutations in the androgen receptor gene are associated with progression of human prostate cancer to androgen-independence. Clin Cancer Res 1996;2:274.

23 Mohler JL, Sharief Y, El-Awady M, Quigley CA, Schalken JA, French FS: Do androgen receptor gene mutations have a role in androgen independent prostatic carcinoma? Presented at the Society of Basic Urology Research, San Antonio, Texas, USA, 1993.

24 Suzuki H, Sato N, Watabe Y, Masai M, Seino S, Shimazaki J: Androgen receptor gene mutations in human prostate cancer. J Steroid Biochem Mol Biol 1993;46:759–765.

25 Castagnaro M, Yandell DW, Dockhorn Dworniczak B, Wolfe HJ, Poremba C: [Androgen receptor gene mutations and p53 gene analysis in advanced prostate cancer]. Verh Dtsch Ges Pathol 1993;77:119–123.
26 Ruizeveld de Winter JA, Janssen PJ, Sleddens HM, Verleun Mooijman MC, Trapman J, Brinkmann AO, Santerse AB, Schröder FH, van der Kwast TH: Androgen receptor status in localized and locally progressive hormone refractory human prostate cancer. Am J Pathol 1994;144:735–746.
27 Gaddipati JP, McLeod DG, Heidenberg HB, Sesterhenn IA, Finger MJ, Moul JW, Srivastava S: Frequent detection of codon 877 mutation in the androgen receptor gene in advanced prostate cancers. Cancer Res 1994;54:2861–2864.
28 Taplin ME, Bubley GJ, Shuster TD, Frantz ME, Spooner AE, Ogata GK, Keer HN, Balk SP: Mutations of the androgen-receptor gene in metastatic androgen-independent prostate cancer. N Engl J Med 1995;332:1393–1398.
29 Tilley WD, Buchanan G, Hickey TE, Horsfall DJ: Detection of androgen receptor gene mutations in human prostate cancers by immunohistochemistry and PCR-SSP (abstract). Proc Am Assoc Cancer Res 1995;36:266.
30 Visakorpi T, Hyytinen E, Koivisto P, Tanner M, Keinanen R, Palmberg C, Palotie A, Tammela T, Isola J, Kallioniemi O: In vivo amplification of the androgen receptor gene and progression of human prostate cancer. Nature Genetics 1995;9:401–406.
31 Scher HI, Liebertz C, Kelly WK, Mazumdar M, Brett C, Schwartz L, Kolvenbag G, Shapario L, Schwartz M: Bicalutamide for advanced prostate cancer: the natural history versus treated history of disease. J Clin Oncol 1997; 15:2928–2938.
32 Joyce R, Fenton MA, Rode P, Constantine M, Gaynes L, Kolvenbag G, DeWolf W, Balk S, Taplin ME, Bubley GJ: High-dose bicalutamide for androgen-independent prostate cancer: effect of prior hormonal therapy. J Urol 1998; 159:149–153.
33 Scher HI, Mazumdar M, Kelly WK: Clinical trials in relapsed prostate cancer: defining the target. J Natl Cancer Inst 1996;88:1623–1634.

European
Urology

F. Debruyne

Department of Urology, University Hospital
Nijmegen, The Netherlands

Introduction

The following papers have arisen from an interactive workshop entitled 'Therapeutic dilemmas in prostate cancer' held at the XIIIth Congress of the European Association of Urology in Barcelona, Spain, 21–25 March 1998. The format of the workshop enabled a lively exchange of information and experiences between the panel members and the audience on some of the issues that face the clinician when deciding which treatments to recommend to prostate cancer patients.

During the first part of the workshop our panel of experts were asked to put forward certain views (not necessarily their own[1]) on treatment choices. Zev Wajsman kindly agreed to present some arguments in favour of combined androgen blockade and the counter arguments were given by Urs Studer. Subsequently Nicholas George discussed the option of watchful waiting, stressing that this needs to be an 'active and progressive supervision policy'. Finally, Martin Gleave explained the rationale behind intermittent androgen suppression as a therapeutic strategy and presented some phase II clinical data on its efficacy. The results from phase III trials are eagerly awaited.

In the second part of the workshop three case histories were presented and the expert panel and audience were asked to vote on which course of action they would recommend during the development of the patients' treatment. These case histories were developed by Hartwig Huland, Nicholas George and myself, and had previously been presented at a similar workshop at the XIIth Congress of the European Association of Urology in Paris, September 1–5, 1996. The results of the comparative voting are discussed in the conclusion to these proceedings.

Prostate cancer continues to dominate everyday urological and oncological practice. The discussion of current dilemmas in the management of prostate cancer continues to challenge our attitudes to therapy.

[1] Please note that each presentation was not a balanced view of a situation as the presenters had been asked to take a particular perspective to support an interesting debate.

KARGER

Fax + 41 61 306 12 34
E-Mail karger@karger.ch
www.karger.com

0302–2838/98/0349–0024$15.00/0

Accessible online at:
http://BioMedNet.com/karger

Prof. Frans Debruyne
426 Department of Urology, University Hospital Nijmegen
Geert Grootplein 10, PO Box 9101
NL–6500 HB Nijmegen (The Netherlands)
Tel. +31 243 613 735, Fax +31 243 541 031

European Urology

Eur Urol 1998;34(suppl 3):25–28

Z. Wajsman

Division of Urology, College of Medicine, University of Gainsville, Fla., USA

Arguments for the Long-Term Use of Combined Androgen Blockade

Key Words
Prostate cancer
Combined androgen blockade
Minimal disease
Luteinizing hormone-releasing hormone agonist
Orchidectomy
Bicalutamide
Flutamide
Nilutamide

Abstract
From what is known about the testicular and adrenal origins of testosterone, and the testosterone dependency of prostate cancer, treatment with combined androgen blockade (CAB) by castration plus an antiandrogen was expected to be beneficial to patients. A number of early studies verified this hypothesis, but the findings needed to be confirmed in large, randomized, prospective studies. Modest but significant benefits of CAB were seen when treatment with leuprorelin plus flutamide was compared with leuprorelin alone. Of note was the increased benefit from CAB seen in patients with minimal metastatic prostate cancer, a finding that needed to be confirmed. A study comparing orchidectomy plus nilutamide with orchidectomy alone showed significant benefits of CAB in terms of time to progression and overall survival. However, a recent major NCI study revealed no benefits for CAB with respect to survival, even for patients with minimal metastatic disease. Results from other clinical studies have been conflicting, perhaps because of the method of castration or differences in antiandrogen used. Before the question of whether CAB significantly benefits patients can be fully answered, a clearer understanding of the interactions between antiandrogens, luteinizing hormone-releasing hormone agonists and receptors, and of the response of prostate cancer to these, is needed.

Historical Background

In 1941, Huggins and Hodges established the fact that prostate cancer is hormone dependent [1]. Approximately 95% of the total testosterone is produced in the testes, with the remainder originating from the adrenal gland – the hypothalamic-pituitary-gonadal axis is well understood. Only 3% of circulating testosterone is unbound and able to enter the prostate cells where it is converted to the active form, dihydrotestosterone (DHT), by 5-α-reductase. DHT is then transported into the nucleus and promotes cell growth. Huggins realized that most patients with prostate cancer demonstrate a dramatic response to androgen withdrawal. Unfortunately, at that time the luxury of the modern mass media was not available and clinical researchers were less 'fame' conscious; it took many years before the hormonal dependency of prostate cancer became widely recognized as benefiting thousands of

KARGER

Fax + 41 61 306 12 34
E-Mail karger@karger.ch
www.karger.com

0302–2838/0349–0025$15.00/0

Accessible online at:
http://BioMedNet.com/karger

Dr. Zev Wajsman
Professor of Surgery, Division of Urology
College of Medicine University of Florida
PO Box 100247, Gainesville, FL 32610-0247 (USA)
Tel. +1 352 392 2501, Fax +1 352 392 8846, E-Mail wajsman@surgery.ufl.edu

Table 1. Median progression-free survival and overall survival in intergroup study 0036 after a follow-up of 42 months [8, 9]

	Median survival (months) [95% CI]	
	progression-free	overall survival
Stage D2 disease		
Leuprorelin 1 mg/day plus flutamide 250 mg tid (n = 303)	16.5 [14.6, 19.5]*	35.6 [31.3, 38.9]**
Leuprorelin 1 mg/day plus placebo (n = 300)	13.9 [11.8, 15.3]	28.3 [25.7, 30.6]
Good performance status and minimal disease [1]		
Leuprorelin plus flutamide (n = 41)	58.3 [NA]	61.0 [NA]
Leuprorelin plus placebo (n = 41)	19.1 [NA]	41.5 [NA]

* p = 0.039 compared with the leuprorelin plus placebo group; ** p = 0.035 compared with the leuprorelin plus placebo group; NA, not available.
1 Involving axial skeleton only and/or one lymph node.

patients, with a Nobel prize for this discovery coming much later.

In 1945 Huggins and Scott [2] suspected that patients who underwent castration may benefit from an adrenalectomy, so removing the only remaining source of testosterone. They, and many others, observed rapid subjective and objective responses although these were all short-lived. Problems with the surgical complications of an adrenalectomy, along with the difficulty of post-operative care, resulted in the loss of interest in this form of combined androgen blockade (CAB). In retrospect it was amazing to see a response in such a poorly selected population – most of these patients had end-stage disease, a large tumour burden and had failed hormone therapy. Today we realize that at least some of the responses could be attributed to the steroid replacement required after adrenalectomy.

In the early 1970s, the discovery of luteinizing hormone-releasing hormone (LH-RH) agonists by Schally and colleagues [3] and the availability of nonsteroidal antiandrogens [4] stimulated interest in modern CAB regimens. Subsequently, Geller's group [5] described the phenomenon of a high concentration of DHT in the prostatic cells of patients who had undergone castration, again suggesting the role of the adrenal gland as a source of testosterone.

Clinical Studies

In 1986, Labrie et al. [6] published the unprecedented results of antiandrogen treatment in patients who failed castration. In 56 patients, an objective response of 43% was reported. In previously untreated patients receiving CAB (n = 88) they reported an objective response of 97%, 30% higher than the historical data on orchidectomy. However, none of the patients had measurable lesions. CAB was widely publicized by this group as a primary treatment for patients who were hormonally naive [7] and their data was widely reported in the non-scientific press, resulting in a massive number of patients moving to Canada for CAB treatment. Some well-conducted clinical trials of CAB followed, but none duplicated these findings. A selection of larger studies of CAB are described below.

Luteinizing Hormone-Releasing Hormone Agonist plus Antiandrogen

In the Intergroup study 0036 in which 603 patients with stage D2 prostate cancer were treated with leuprorelin plus flutamide or leuprorelin alone, modest, but clinically and statistically significant, benefits in terms of time to disease progression (p = 0.039) and overall survival (p = 0.035) were seen with CAB (table 1) [8]. In addition, for a subgroup of 82 patients with minimal disease, the median time to progression was 58.3 months for patients receiving CAB compared with 19.1 months for the placebo group, a difference of 39.2 months (table 1) [9]. Overall survival in this minimal disease subgroup was 20 months longer in the CAB group compared with the placebo group. The number of patients with minimal metastatic prostate cancer at first presentation is increasing, mainly because of greater awareness and earlier diagnosis of prostate cancer through annual screening by measurement of PSA serum concentrations. Therefore, CAB may be of particular benefit in this expanding population.

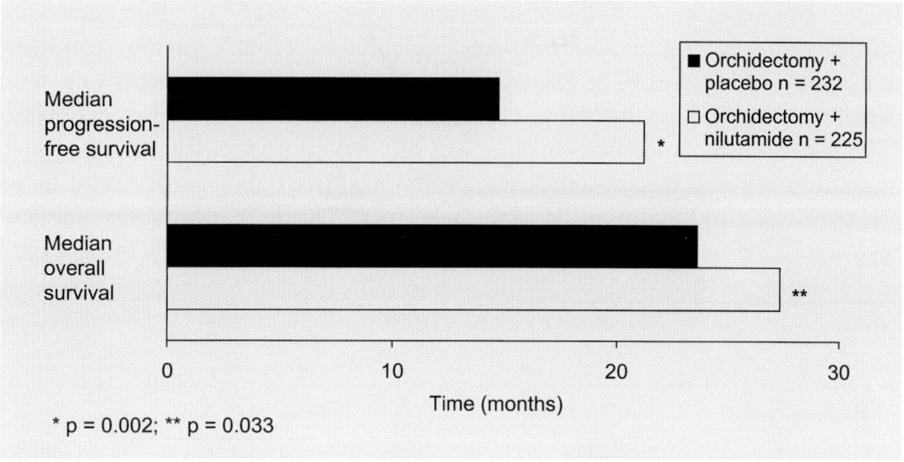

Fig. 1. An increased median time to progression and overall survival is seen with combined androgen blockade (orchidectomy plus nilutamide) compared with orchidectomy alone. Adapted with permission [12].

When LH-RH agonists are given as monotherapy two factors need to be taken into account: patient compliance and the 'flare' effect which is caused by an initial surge in testosterone levels. In CAB with an LH-RH agonist, any benefit compared with monotherapy may be due to prevention of the flare effect by the antiandrogen component. The flare effect does not occur after orchidectomy, so studies with CAB using orchidectomy and an antiandrogen would give a clearer indication of the benefits of CAB.

Orchidectomy Plus Antiandrogen

In a large international study (Intergroup study 0105), 1,371 patients with stage D2 prostate cancer were treated with orchidectomy alone or orchidectomy plus flutamide [10]. After 8 years of study and a follow-up of 4 years, there was only 1 month difference (31 versus 30 months) in median survival for the CAB group compared with the orchidectomy plus placebo group. The progression-free survival was 21 months in the orchidectomy plus flutamide group and 18 months in the orchidectomy alone group. Neither of these differences were statistically significant. Patient well-being was affected by this antiandrogen; there was a 3.3% incidence of diarrhoea in the orchidectomy plus flutamide group compared with 0.8% in the orchidectomy plus placebo group [10]. Interestingly, the reduction in serum PSA concentrations was greater in the CAB group with no effect on survival, questioning the validity of a PSA response to flutamide as an indicator of success.

In contrast to the NCI study, clear benefits with CAB were demonstrated in an international study of 457 patients with stage D2 prostate cancer comparing orchidectomy plus nilutamide with orchidectomy plus placebo [11, 12]. After a follow-up period of 8.5 years a significant difference in median progression-free survival was seen between the groups, time to progression being 21.2 months in the CAB group compared with 14.7 months in the orchidectomy alone group ($p = 0.002$) (fig. 1) [12]. The overall survival was 27.3 months in the CAB group and 23.6 months in the orchidectomy alone group ($p = 0.033$) (fig. 1). Nilutamide was well tolerated with the two most frequent adverse events, hot flushes and transient disturbance, seen in 28% and 27% of patients in the CAB group, and 22% and 3% in the orchidectomy group, respectively [11]. There was no increase in the incidence of adverse events with longer exposure to nilutamide [12]. Early normalisation of PSA concentration predicted improved long-term response to hormonal treatment [12].

Conclusion

Clearly we do not have a complete understanding of the biology of prostate cancer in relation to its hormonal dependency. Not all clinical trials demonstrate a benefit for patients receiving CAB [13]; these inconsistent results may be explained by, for example, the substantial difference between surgical and medical castration and the role of LH-RH, antiandrogen receptors and their stimulation or suppression. Also, significant PSA reduction does not necessarily lead to increased survival and therefore studies must have a sufficiently long follow-up period to demonstrate efficacy. Finally, antiandrogens prevent the disease flare that occurs with LH-RH agonists so results with medical or surgical castration as part of CAB may differ.

In deciding whether CAB benefits patients we must take into account that not all antiandrogens are equal in terms of efficacy and tolerability. The results from a study that directly compared bicalutamide and flutamide as part of CAB indicate that specific combinations of CAB components that are effective and better tolerated, such as LH-RH agonists and bicalutamide, will make this treatment regimen a clearer option [14, 15].

Further basic research is needed into the role of the various antiandrogens available, their receptors and their interactions with LH-RH agonists. Until then clinical studies can not be rationally designed to clarify the conflicting results obtained to date. In the future our clearer understanding of the biological mechanisms involved in prostate cancer will enable antiandrogens to have a significant impact on the clinical management of patients.

References

1 Huggins C, Hodges CV: Studies on prostate cancer. 1. The effect of castration, of estrogen and of androgen injection on serum phospatases in metastatic carcinoma of the prostate. Cancer Res 1941;1:293–297.

2 Huggins C, Scott WW: Bilateral adrenalectomy in prostate cancer. Ann Surg 1945;122:1031–1041.

3 Schally AV, Arimura A, Baba Y, Nair RM, Matsuo H, Redding TW, Debeljuk L: Isolation and properties of the FSH and LH-releasing hormone. Biochem Biophys Res Commun 1971;43:393–399.

4 Neri R, Florance K, Koziol P, Van Cleave S: A biological profile of nonsteroidal antiandrogen, SCH 13521 (4′-nitro-3′-trifluoromethylisobutyranilide). Endocrinology 1972;91:427–437.

5 Geller J, De La Vega DJ, Albert JD, Nachtscheim DA: Tissue dihydrotestosterone levels and clinical response to hormonal therapy. I. Patients with advanced prostate cancer. J Clin Endocrinol Metab 1984;58:36–40.

6 Labrie F, Dupont A, Bélanger A, St-Arnaud R, Giguère M, Lacourcière Y, Edmonde J, Monfette G: Treatment of prostate cancer with gonadotropin-releasing hormone agonists. Endocr Rev 1986;7:67–74.

7 Labrie F, Bélanger A, Simard J, Labrie C, Dupont A: Combination therapy for prostate cancer. Endocrine and biologic basis of its choice as new standard first-line therapy. Cancer 1993;71(suppl 3):1059–1067.

8 Crawford ED, Eisenberger MA, McLeod DG, Spaulding JT, Benson R, Dorr FA, Blumenstein BA, Davis MA, Goodman PJ: A controlled trial of leuprolide with and without flutamide in prostate carcinoma. N Engl J Med 1989;321:419–424.

9 Daneshgari F, Crawford ED: Endocrine therapy for advanced carcinoma of the prostate. Cancer 1993;71(suppl 3):1089–1097.

10 Crawford ED, Eisenberger MA, McLeod DG, Wilding G, Blumenstein BA: Comparison of bilateral orchiectomy with or without flutamide for the treatment of patients with stage D2 adenocarcinoma of the prostate: results of NCI intergroup study 0105 (SWOG and ECOG). J Urol 1997;157(suppl):336 (Abs 1311).

11 Janknegt RA, Abbou CC, Bartoletti R, Bernstein-Hahn L, Bracken B, Brisset JM, Calais Da Siva F, Chisholm G, Crawford ED, Debruyne FMJ, Dijkman GD, Frick J, Goedhals L, Knönagel H, Venner PM: Orchiectomy and nilutamide or placebo as treatment of metastatic prostatic cancer in a multinational double-blind randomized trial. J Urol 1993;149:77–83.

12 Dijkman GA, Janknegt RA, de Reijke TM, Debruyne FMJ for the International Anandron Study Group: Long-term efficacy and safety of nilutamide plus castration in advanced prostate cancer, and the significance of early prostate specific antigen normalization. J Urol 1997;158:160–163.

13 Studer UE, Mills RD: Arguments against the long-term use of combined androgen blockade. Eur Urol 1998;34(suppl 3):29–32.

14 Schellhammer PF, Sharifi R, Block NL, Soloway MS, Venner PM, Patterson AL, Sarosdy MF, Vogelzang NJ, Schellenger JJ, Kolvenbag GJCM, for the Casodex Combination Study Group: Clinical benefits of bicalutamide compared with flutamide in combined androgen blockade for patients with advanced prostatic carcinoma: final report of a double-blind, randomized, multicenter trial. Urology 1997;50:330–336.

15 Sarosdy MF, Schellhammer PF, Sharifi R, Block NL, Soloway MS, Venner PM, Patterson AL, Vogelzang NJ, Chodack GW, Klein EA, Schellenger JJ, Kolvenbag GJCM: Comparison of goserelin and leuprolide in combined androgen blockade therapy. Urology 1998;52:82–88.

European Urology

Eur Urol 1998;34(suppl 3):29–32

U.E. Studer
R.D. Mills

Department of Urology,
University of Berne, Switzerland

Arguments against the Long-Term Use of Combined Androgen Blockade

Key Words
Combined androgen blockade
Antiandrogen
Luteinizing hormone-releasing hormone agonist
Orchiectomy
Prostate cancer

Abstract
Androgen deprivation therapy is the most effective systemic treatment for advanced prostate cancer. However, as most patients who die from prostate cancer have hormone refractory disease, fine tuning of antiandrogen treatment by combined androgen blockade (CAB) can not be expected to improve survival significantly. Only the South West Oncology Intergroup (SWOG) study 0036 has shown a significant advantage for CAB compared with luteinizing hormone-releasing hormone (LH-RH) agonist alone. However, the results of this study should be interpreted with caution as the patients had to self-administer their treatment by daily injection so compliance may not have been optimal. Also, those receiving LH-RH agonist alone were not covered against disease flare. Indeed, no trial using depot LH-RH agonist with or without flutamide has been able to show a survival benefit. When treatment with LH-RH agonist plus antiandrogen was compared with orchiectomy alone, only the European Organization for Research and Treatment of Cancer (EORTC) study 30853 showed a significant difference in favour of CAB. However, in this study an increased proportion of patients receiving CAB may have had a more favourable prognosis. Only one study comparing orchiectomy plus antiandrogen with orchiectomy alone has shown an advantage for CAB therapy, and this was only slight. Therefore, as yet there is no justification for long-term use of CAB. However, short-term antiandrogen treatment must be used to prevent disease flare during initiation of LH-RH agonist treatment.

Introduction

Seventy years after its addition to the urological therapeutic armamentarium, androgen deprivation therapy is still the most effective systemic treatment for advanced prostate cancer. However, those patients who die from prostate cancer die from hormone refractory disease. Therefore, although monotherapy with luteinizing hormone-releasing hormone (LH-RH) agonists or antiandrogens have a place in the management of prostate cancer, fine tuning of antiandrogen treatment by combined androgen blockade (CAB) would not be expected to make

KARGER

Fax + 41 61 306 12 34
E-Mail karger@karger.ch
www.karger.com

0302–2838/98/0349–0029$15.00/0

Accessible online at:
http://BioMedNet.com/karger

Dr. Urs E. Studer
Department of Urology, University of Berne
Inselspital – Anna Seiler-Haus
CH–3010 Berne (Switzerland)
Tel +41 31 632 3621, Fax +41 31 632 2180

Table 1. Randomized trials of luteinizing hormone-releasing hormone agonist alone or with antiandrogen

Combined treatment	Control	No. patients	Survival	Ref.
Leuprorelin + flutamide	Leuprorelin + placebo	603	$p = 0.035$	1
Goserelin + flutamide	Goserelin	571	NS	2
Goserelin + flutamide	Goserelin	373	NS	3
Goserelin + CPA	Goserelin	349	NS	4
Leuprorelin + nilutamide	Leuprorelin + placebo	333	NS	5
Goserelin + CPA	Goserelin	328	NS	6
Goserelin + flutamide	Goserelin + placebo	245	NS	7

CPA, cyproterone acetate; NS, not significant.
Adapted with permission [8].

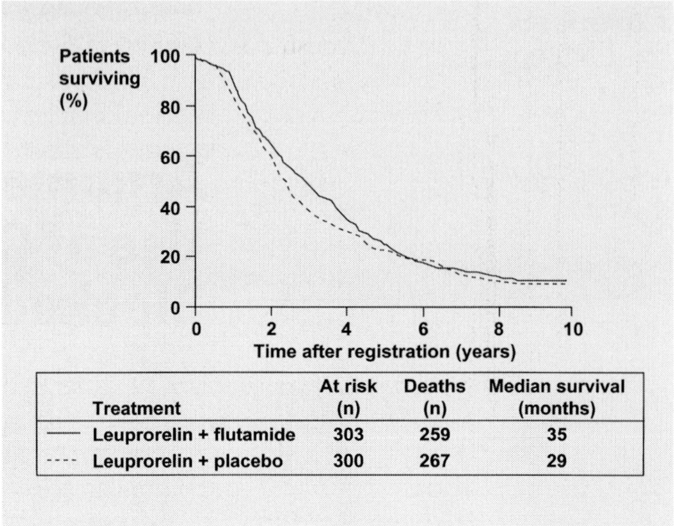

Fig. 1. Overall survival in patients receiving leuprorelin plus flutamide compared with leuprorelin plus placebo. Results from April 20, 1995 update of NCI intergroup protocol 0036. Adapted with permission [10].

a major difference to survival, even when the androgens of adrenal origin are suppressed. This has been confirmed by prospective, randomized trials as discussed below.

Luteinizing Hormone-Releasing Hormone Agonists plus Antiandrogens

Little improvement in survival rates has been demonstrated in prospective randomized trials comparing LH-RH agonists with or without antiandrogens (table 1) [1–8]. Only the South West Oncology Intergroup (SWOG) study 0036 showed a significant advantage in favour of combined androgen blockade (CAB) [1]; the authors must be credited for having undertaken this study in the early 1980s. Although a large number of patients were enrolled, there are many reasons not to over-interpret the survival benefit.

- The difference in median survival had a low statistical power. In more recent updates of this study, no p values were published [9, 10] (fig. 1).
- If the difference in survival was real, the patients in the LH-RH agonist only group may have died earlier because of disease flare.
- The LH-RH agonist had to be self-administered by daily subcutaneous injections. Therefore, patient compliance may have been a problem. No serum testosterone measurements were done to confirm castrate levels were reached. If patients recommenced interrupted treatment, the risk of disease flare would be several fold higher.
- All similar studies using a depot LH-RH agonist where compliance was not an issue showed no survival difference in favour of long-term, combined treatment.

Luteinizing Hormone-Releasing Hormone Agonists plus Antiandrogen versus Orchiectomy

Of three studies comparing LH-RH agonists plus antiandrogen with orchiectomy alone (table 2) [11–13], only the European Organization for Research and Treatment of Cancer (EORTC) study 30853 showed a significant difference in favour of the combined treatment group [11]. Subgroup analysis showed that the survival difference resulted from patients with a good prognosis. Unfortunately, analysis of the treatment groups according to risk factors showed that the combined treatment group contained patients at lower risk despite proper randomization, although the small number of patients meant that this did not reach a statistically significant level. In contrast, the patients in the orchiectomy group more frequently had a poor performance status, cardiovascular disease, pre-treatment weight loss and advanced disease compared with those in the LH-RH agonist plus flutamide group [14, 15]. In the Danish Prostate Cancer Group study, which had a similar number of patients from the same area of Europe as the patients in the EORTC study 30853, improved survival for CAB therapy when compared with orchiectomy alone was not demonstrated [13].

Orchiectomy plus Antiandrogens

Of all studies comparing orchiectomy with or without an antiandrogen (table 3) [16–22] only one showed a benefit for CAB, with a slight survival advantage of 3 months in patients who received orchiectomy plus nilutamide [17]. This possible survival advantage needs to be confirmed by a second, independent study before treatment guidelines can recommend orchiectomy plus nilutamide as standard treatment. Moreover, as presented by Crawford at the American Urological Association (AUA) meeting in 1997, the large Intergroup study 0105 comparing orchiectomy plus flutamide with orchiectomy plus placebo in 1,378 patients showed no survival advantage for either treatment [16]. Thus, any advantage seen with the addition of an antiandrogen is not necessarily true across the class. In this study, time to prostate-specific antigen (PSA) progression was significantly longer in the patients treated with CAB. This substantiates earlier findings that flutamide may decrease PSA secretion, without necessarily killing the prostate cancer cells or prolonging survival [23].

The Place of Antiandrogens in Prostate Cancer Therapy

As there is no convincing evidence for a significant improvement in survival when long-term flutamide treatment is added to either orchiectomy or LH-RH agonist depot treatment, and as flutamide has side effects (including gastrointestinal disturbances and hepatotoxicity), there is no justification for giving long-term CAB with flutamide apart from in prospective randomized studies. Although bicalutamide appears to have a better side-effect profile than flutamide [24], no results have shown that it is significantly more effective than flutamide in terms of survival, or that androgen receptor adaptation causing tumour stimulation will not occur. However, antiandrogens are useful when given before and during initiation of LH-RH agonist depot treatment to prevent disease flare.

Table 2. Randomized trials of combined androgen blockade compared with orchiectomy

Combined treatment	Control	No. patients	Survival	Ref.
Goserelin + flutamide	Orchiectomy	326	p = 0.04	11
Buserelin + CPA	Orchiectomy	302	NS	12
Goserelin + flutamide	Orchiectomy	262	NS	13

CPA, cyproterone acetate; NS, not significant.
Adapted with permission [8].

Table 3. Randomized trials of orchiectomy alone or with antiandrogen

Combined treatment	Control	No. patients	Survival	Ref.
Orchiectomy + flutamide	Orchiectomy + placebo	1,380	NS	16
Orchiectomy + nilutamide	Orchiectomy + placebo	457	p = 0.013	17
Orchiectomy + CPA	Orchiectomy	221	NS	18
Orchiectomy + flutamide	Orchiectomy + placebo	216	NS	19
Orchiectomy + nilutamide	Orchiectomy + placebo	194	NS	20
Orchiectomy + nilutamide	Orchiectomy + placebo	127	NS	21
Orchiectomy + nilutamide	Orchiectomy + placebo	125	NS	22

CPA, cyproterone acetate; NS, not significant.
Adapted with permission [8].

Conclusion

Androgen deprivation therapy is an effective treatment for prostate cancer, but there is no evidence that fine tuning by the addition of antiandrogens in CAB improves survival to a significant extent. Nevertheless, antiandrogens must be used in short-term treatment to prevent disease flare.

References

1 Crawford ED, Eisenberger MA, McLeod DG, Spaulding JT, Benson R, Dorr FA, Blumenstein BA, Davis MA, Goodman PJ: A controlled clinical trial of leuprolide with and without flutamide in prostatic carcinoma. N Engl J Med 1989;321:419–424.

2 Tyrrell CJ, Altwein JE, Klippel F, Varenhorst E, Lunglmayr G, Boccardo F, Holdaway IM, Haefliger JM, Jordaan JP: A multicenter randomized trial comparing the luteinizing hormone-releasing hormone analogue goserelin acetate alone and with flutamide in the treatment of advanced prostate cancer. The International Prostate Cancer Study Group. J Urol 1991;146:1321–1326.

3 Boccardo F, Pace M, Rubagotti A, Guarneri D, Decensi A, Oneto F, Martorana G, Giuliani L, Selvaggi F, Battaglia M, Delli Ponti U, Petracco S, Cortellini P, Ziveri M, Ferraris V, Bruttini GP, Epis R, Comeri G, Gallo G, and other participants in the Italian Prostatic Cancer Project (PONCAP) Study Group: Goserelin acetate with or without flutamide in the treatment of patients with locally advanced or metastatic prostate cancer. Eur J Cancer 1993;29A: 1088–1093.

4 Brewster SF, Gillatt DA, Chadwick D, Gingell JC, British Prostate Cancer Study Group: A randomised controlled trial of the LHRH analogue Zoladex versus cyproterone acetate versus a combination of the two in metastatic carcinoma of the prostate. In Tenth Congress of the European Association of Urology, Genoa, July 22–25, 1992.

5 Crawford ED, Smith JA, Soloway MS, Lange PH, Lynch DF, Al-Juburi A, Bracken RB, Heyden N, Bertagna C: Treatment of stage D2 prostate cancer with leuprolide and anandron compared to leuprolide and placebo; in Murphy G, et al (eds): Recent Advances in Urological Cancer Diagnosis and Treatment. Diagnostic and Therapeutic Progress in Urological Cancers. Paris, FIIS, 1990.

6 Di Silverio F, Serio M, D'Eramo G, Sciarra F: Zoladex vs Zoladex plus cyproterone acetate in the treatment of advanced prostatic cancer: a multicenter Italian study. Eur Urol 1990;18 (suppl 3):54–61.

7 Fourcade RO, Cariou G, Coloby P, Colombel P, Coulange C, Grise P, Mangin P, Soret JY, Poterre M: Total androgen blockade with Zoladex plus flutamide vs Zoladex alone in advanced prostatic carcinoma: interim report of a multicenter, double-blind, placebo-controlled study. Eur Urol 1990;18(suppl 3):45–47.

8 Denis L: Commentary on maximal androgen blockade in prostate cancer: a theory to put into practice? Prostate 1995;27:233–240.

9 Crawford ED: Challenges in the management of prostate cancer. Br J Urol 1992;70(suppl 1): 33–38.

10 DeAntoni E, Crawford ED: Neuere Multicenter Studienprotokolle in den USA für Patienten mit einem metastasierten Prostatakarzinom. [Recent multicentre study protocols in the USA for patients with metastatic prostatic carcinoma.] Urologe A 1995;34:382–388.

11 Denis LJ, Keuppens F, Smith PH, Whelan P, Carneiro de Moura JL, Newling D, Bono A, Sylvester R for the EORTC Genito-Urinary Tract Cancer Cooperative Group and the EORTC Data Center: Maximal androgen blockade: final analysis of EORTC phase III trial 30853. Eur Urol 1998;33:144–151.

12 De Voogt HJ, Studer U, Schröder FH, Klein JG, de Pauw M, Sylvester R: Maximum androgen blockade (MAB), using LHR-agonist buserelin in combination with short-term (2 weeks) or long-term (continuously) cyproterone-acetate (CPA), is not superior to standard androgen deprivation in the treatment of advanced prostate cancer. Final analysis of EORTC GU group trial 30843. Eur Urol 1998;33:152–158.

13 Iversen P, Christensen MG, Friis E, Hornbol P, Hvidt V, Iversen HG, Klarskov P, Krarup T, Lund F, Mogensen P, Pedersen T, Rasmussen F, Rose C, Skaarup P, Wolf H: A phase III trial of Zoladex and flutamide versus orchiectomy in the treatment of patients with advanced carcinoma of the prostate. Cancer 1990;66(suppl): 1058–1066.

14 Denis LJ, Carniero de Moura JL, Bono A, Sylvester R, Whelan P, Newling D, de Pauw M, on behalf of the EORTC GU Group and EORTC Data Center: Goserelin acetate and flutamide versus bilateral orchiectomy: a phase III EORTC trial (30853). Urology 1993;42:119–129.

15 Newling DW, Denis L, Vermeylen K: Orchiectomy versus goserelin and flutamide in the treatment of newly diagnosed metastatic prostate cancer. Analysis of the criteria of evaluation used in the European Organization for Research and Treatment of Cancer – Genitourinary Group Study 30853. Cancer 1993; 72(suppl 12):3793–3798.

16 Crawford ED, Eisenberger MA, McLeod DG, Wilding G, Blumenstein BA: Comparison of bilateral orchiectomy with or without flutamide for the treatment of patients (PTS) with stage D2 adenocarcinoma of the prostate: results of NCI Intergroup Study 0105 (SWOG and ECOG). J Urol 1997;157:336(A1311).

17 Dijkman GA, Janknegt RA, de Reijke TM, Debruyne FMJ: Long-term efficacy and safety of nilutamide plus castration in advanced prostate cancer, and the significance of early prostate specific antigen normalization. J Urol 1997;153:160–163.

18 Robinson MR: A further analysis of European Organization for Research and Treatment of Cancer protocol 30805. Orchidectomy versus orchidectomy plus cyproterone acetate versus low-dose diethylstilbestrol. Cancer 1993;72 (suppl):3855–3857.

19 Zalcberg JR, Raghaven D, Marshall V, Thompson PJ: Bilateral orchidectomy and flutamide versus orchidectomy alone in newly diagnosed patients with metastatic carcinoma of the prostate: an Australian multicentre trial. Br J Urol 1996;77:865–869.

20 Béland G, Elhilali M, Fradet Y, Laroche B, Ramsey EW, Trachtenberg J, Venner PM, Tewari HD: A controlled trial of castration with and without nilutamide in metastatic prostatic carcinoma. Cancer 1990;66(suppl 5):1074–1079.

21 Brisset JM, Bertagna C, Fiet J, de Géry A, Hucher M, Husson JM, Tremblay D, Raynaud JP: Total androgen blockade vs orchiectomy in stage D prostate cancer. Preliminary results of a multicentre French trial; in Klijn JGM, et al (eds): Hormonal Manipulation of Cancer. Peptides, Growth Factors, and New (Anti) Steroidal Agents. New York, Raven Press, 1987.

22 Namer M, Toubol J, Caty A, Couette JE, Douchez J, Kerbrat P, Droz JP: A randomized double-blind study evaluating Anandron associated with orchiectomy in stage D prostate cancer. J Steroid Biochem Mol Biol 1990;37:909–915.

23 Young CY, Montgomery BT, Andrews PE, Qui SD, Bilhartz DL, Tindall DJ: Hormonal regulation of prostate-specific antigen messenger RNA in human prostatic adenocarcinoma cell line LNCaP. Cancer Res 1991;51:3748–3752.

24 Schellhammer PF, Sharifi R, Block NL, Soloway MS, Venner PM, Patterson AL, Sarosdy MF, Vogelzang NJ, Schellenger JJ, Kolvenbag GJ, on behalf of the Casodex Combination Study Group: Clinical benefits of bicalutamide compared with flutamide in combined androgen blockade for patients with advanced prostatic carcinoma: final report of a double-blind, randomized, multicenter trial. Urology 1997; 50:330–336.

European Urology

Eur Urol 1998;34(suppl 3):33–36

N. George

Department of Urology, Withington Hospital, University of Manchester, UK

Therapeutic Dilemmas in Prostate Cancer: Justification for Watchful Waiting

Key Words
Watchful waiting
Prostate cancer

Abstract
Despite the large numbers of elderly men known to harbour pathological evidence of prostate cancer and evidence from observational studies suggesting the prolonged time course of such disease, conservative management of such patients has not enjoyed the widespread support of urologists, particularly in the USA, where monitoring of patients is often dismissed as 'intentional neglect' rather than 'watchful waiting'. This paper outlines the rationale and principles underlying expectant treatment of patients with prostate cancer.

Biological Principles

Classical post-mortem studies [1] show that prostate cancer is most commonly diagnosed in the elderly, a trend which has continued [2] with the advent of widespread prostate-specific antigen (PSA) testing by primary physicians and gerontologists. Observational studies [3, 4] have clearly demonstrated that for patients with well differentiated tumours, time to progression may be particularly prolonged, presumably because of slow tumour doubling time (fig. 1). Thus, for those whose biological life expectancy is not likely to exceed this figure, treatment – usually hormonal manipulation in the older age group – carries a greater burden of morbidity than does the primary disease. The same arguments cannot be used for poorly differentiated tumours which are likely to cause death of the patient at any age, while the behaviour of moderately differentiated tumours remains open to question. In the author's experience moderately differentiated lesions tend to parallel the clinical course of patients with poorly rather than well differentiated histology.

In practical terms, watchful waiting is most applicable to the 'average' older patient (aged more than 70 years), with well differentiated pathology and 'average' life expectancy. It is certainly not suitable for any patient aged less than 65 years with disease curable by radical therapy unless the patient has limited life expectancy for any other reason (i.e. cardiac or vascular disease). Between the ages of 65 and 70 years careful clinical judgement is required, but more often than not radical therapy will be chosen for those with disease of appropriate early stage. Younger patients (aged less than 70 years) with disease that is not curable by radical treatment (ie, T3NXMO) may be offered watchful waiting but, as stated above, it is likely that the disease process will advance and lead to death. The timing and nature of therapeutic intervention in such patients remains open to debate.

Assuming a patient has no bone metastases at the time of diagnosis, the fundamental principle of watchful waiting is to avoid bone scan conversion at all costs. Patients with slowly growing primary lesions or disease in lymph nodes rarely have major symptomatic problems and such

KARGER

Fax + 41 61 306 12 34
E-Mail karger@karger.ch
www.karger.com

0302–2838/0349–0033$15.00/0

Accessible online at:
http://BioMedNet.com/karger

Dr. Nick George
Department of Urology
Withington Hospital, University of Manchester
West Didsbury, M20 2CR (UK)
Tel. +44 161 291 3766, Fax +44 161 291 3767

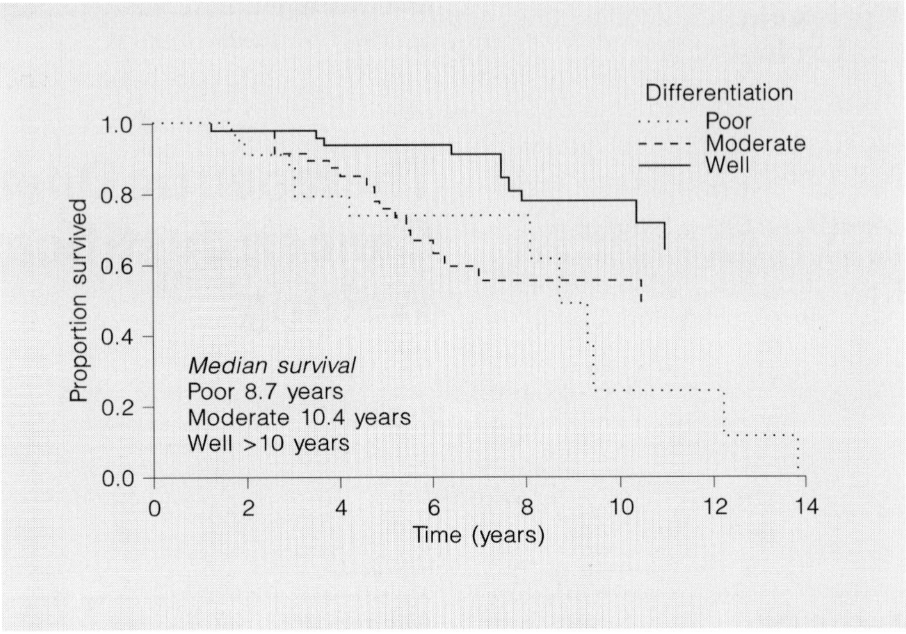

Fig. 1. Survival of patients with localized (bone scan negative) prostate cancer by initial histological classification (1980–1995). Unpublished follow-up data from patients originally studied and reported [3]. Median survival for those with well differentiated tumours has not yet been reached.

difficulties are usually overcome by simple outflow tract surgery or other minor interventions. Occasionally prostate cancer may manifest by relatively massive nodal enlargement but even this degree of disease, in the absence of any bony secondaries, may carry a significantly better prognosis [5] than patients who present with disease in bone which is both painful and relapses soon after treatment.

The precise reason for rapid disease progression of patients with bony metastases remains unclear. It is possible that interaction between resorbing osteoclasts and tumour cells, perhaps mediated by locally active growth factors or cytokines, leads to paracrine-like stimulation which is relatively resistant to external modulation (i.e. hormonal manipulation). Studies of active tumour in human bone have shown that antiosteoclast agents may suppress osteoclast activity in normal bone but fail to prevent resorption in areas adjacent to tumour deposits, suggesting continuing local interactive stimulation [6].

Before the advent of PSA testing only acid phosphatase and repeated bone scans were available to those wishing to pursue a watchful waiting policy which thus often failed to predict osseous metastases. Since then a number of studies have disclosed the range of PSA within which it is relatively safe to reassure the patient on a surveillance programme [7]. Nonetheless, PSA may be a poor surrogate marker for tumour activity and although most watchful waiting protocols will involve patients with well differentiated neoplasms, tumour grade may deteriorate with time so due vigilance will always be required. Levels of PSA (Hybritech) approaching 50 ng (fig. 2) will be an indication that urgent treatment should be considered to prevent bone scan conversion.

Psychological Aspects of Watchful Waiting

It cannot be emphasised often enough that watchful waiting is an *active* process and not a licence for dismissal and neglect – 'come back if you experience bone pain'. The surgeon will need to explain carefully to both the patient and his family the nature of a watchful waiting policy, the scientific basis underpinning the regimen and the exact nature of the follow-up protocol. This is never a task to be delegated to junior doctors – the patient and his family must have confidence that the surgeon understands the tumour biology and will be vigilant with regard to PSA testing which ideally should be at no greater than 6-month intervals. In summary, the patient must be confident that the watchful waiting policy will allow him a significant period of life free of treatment side effects but that if treatment is necessary it will be anticipated and carried out in good time. Such confidence allows many older men the chance to live out their natural lives without the need for castration or other forms of hormonal manipulation.

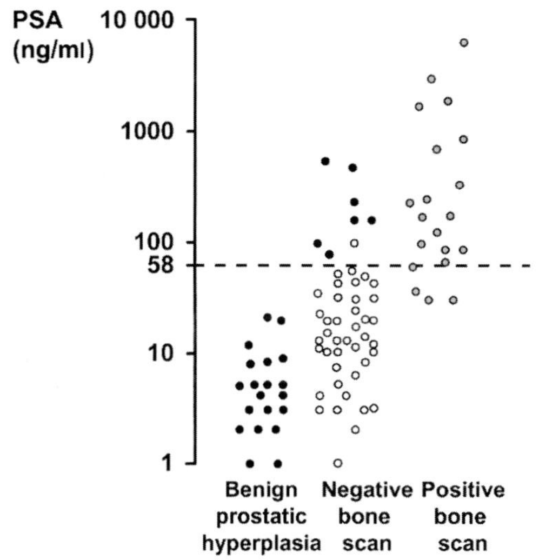

Fig. 2. PSA values in patients with untreated prostate cancer reported. Open circles in patients with negative bone scan – acid phosphatase raised above normal levels suggesting occult bony metastases (– – –): optimum cut off level of PSA for metastatic disease in bone. Adapted with permission [7].

Watchful Waiting in Patients Aged Less than 65 Years

As stated above, watchful waiting is generally not suited to patients with curable or locally advanced disease with negative bone scans. Nevertheless, it has to be conceded that some of these patients discovered by PSA testing might have tumours of such low bioactivity that they might survive unscathed into older age. It is at present impossible to distinguish these patients from the majority who will progress so it is accepted by most authorities [8] that a degree of over-treatment has to be tolerated for younger men with early prostate cancer. Because of this doubt some patients may refuse treatment; regular PSA testing may help in these patients but they should understand that by the time the biopotential of the tumour has declared itself, the disease may have moved from curable to incurable by radical local therapy.

Who Should Be Treated?

In summary, active treatment should be offered to younger patients with potentially curable disease, regardless of grade. The poor prognosis (fig. 1) of those with poorly differentiated lesions should also lead to serious consideration of active radical therapy, even in the older patient. Moderately differentiated histology, in the author's experience, should to a degree tip the scales in favour of more radical treatment at any particular age. Patients with incurable local disease (T3NXMO) may opt for watchful waiting for an unspecified (but highly supervised) period but are, sooner or later, likely to require therapeutic intervention by hormonal manipulation.

The MRC Trial of Deferred Treatment [9]

Published in 1997, the MRC trial has caused considerable comment among urologists. Although a number of valuable lessons were learnt from this study, it is acknowledged that there are a number of questions arising from its design and conclusions. In particular, trial recruitment was prolonged with some variation in entry criteria, and a large number of surgeons admitted small numbers of patients. Of particular concern was the fact that 29 patients died of prostate cancer without any treatment being offered. Although many of these cases might have had good reason for not receiving therapy, the given impression of the trial appears to contrast markedly with the principles of active vigilance described above.

This point is further emphasised by analysing the patients who presented initially with a negative bone scan. The trial was active between 1985 and 1993 and thus through much of this period the sensitive PSA measurements should have been available to those advocating deferred treatment. Despite this, 144 patients progressed from negative to positive bone scan on surveillance leading to significant levels of pain or other skeletal complications. It may be concluded that lack of PSA follow-up data in the M0 group determines that much of the study is of historical interest only.

The trial also addressed the particular case of the patient with bone metastases who has no symptoms referable to his disease. There has indeed been a school of thought that treatment should be withheld from such patients on the grounds that their situation cannot be improved; manipulation can be reserved for the time when it is needed. The trial showed reasonably convincingly that the incidence of complications (i.e. spinal collapse) was greater in the deferred treatment group and hence the usual policy of immediate treatment of the newly diagnosed patient with M1 disease (symptomatic or otherwise) was deemed to be correct.

Conclusion

In summary, watchful waiting is seen to be an active and progressive supervision policy for certain patient groups with specific forms of prostatic neoplasia defined by both stage and grade of disease. Adherence to these accepted protocols may offer significant benefit to the patient, his family and to the attending surgeon as long as he is prepared to follow a policy of vigilant surveillance.

References

1 Franks LM: Aetiology, epidemiology and pathology of prostate cancer. Cancer 1973;323:1092–1095.
2 CRC Fact Sheet 20.4. Cancer Research Campaign, London, 1994.
3 George NJR: Natural history of localised prostatic cancer managed by conservative therapy alone. Lancet 1988;1:494–497.
4 Adolfsson J, Rönström L, Carstensen J, Lowhagen T, Hedlund PO: The natural course of low stage, low grade prostatic carcinoma. Br J Urol 1990;65:611–614.
5 Sandhu DPS, Mayor PE, Sambrook P, George NJR: Increased survival of patients with massive lymphadenopathy and prostate cancer: evidence of heterogeneous tumour behaviour. Br J Urol 1990;66:415–419.
6 Clarke NW, McClure J, George NJR: Disodium pamidronate identifies differential osteoclastic bone resorption in metastatic prostate cancer. Br J Urol 1992;69:64–70.
7 Pantelides ML, Bowman SP, George NJR: Levels of prostatic specific antigen that predicts skeletal spread in prostate cancer. Br J Urol 1992;70:299–303.
8 Schröder FH: To screen or not to screen. Br Med J 1993;306:407–408.
9 MRC Prostate Cancer Working Party Investigators Group: Immediate versus deferred treatment for advanced prostatic cancer: initial results of the MRC trial. Br J Urol 1997;79:235–246.

European Urology

Eur Urol 1998;34(suppl 3):37–41

M. Gleave
N. Bruchovsky
S.L. Goldenberg
P. Rennie

Division of Urology, Vancouver General Hospital, University of British Columbia, Vancouver, Canada

Intermittent Androgen Suppression for Prostate Cancer: Rationale and Clinical Experience

Key Words
Intermittent androgen suppression
Androgen independent
Androgen ablation
Quality of life
Prostate cancer

Abstract
The rationale behind intermittent androgen suppression (IAS) is based on: (1) observations that androgen ablation is palliative, not curative, in most patients with prostate cancer, and that quality of life must be considered; (2) the assumption that immediate androgen ablation is superior to delayed therapy in improving survival; (3) the hypothesis that if tumour cells surviving androgen withdrawal are forced into a normal pathway of differentiation by androgen replacement, then apoptotic potential might be restored and progression to androgen independence delayed. Several centres have now tested the feasibility of IAS therapy in non-randomized groups of prostate cancer patients using serum of prostate-specific antigen levels as trigger points. Clinical data suggest that prostate cancer is amenable to control by IAS and offers clinicians an opportunity to improve patients' quality of life by balancing the benefits of immediate androgen ablation (delayed progression and prolonged survival) while reducing treatment-related side effects and expense. Whether time to progression and survival is affected in a beneficial or adverse way is being studied in randomized, prospective protocols.

Introduction

Surgical or medical castration results in a median progression-free survival of 12–33 months and a median overall survival of 23–37 months in patients with stage D2 prostate cancer [1]. However, for reasons that remain undefined, the apoptotic process induced by androgen ablation fails to eliminate the entire malignant cell population, and after a variable period of time averaging 24 months, progression inevitably occurs with increasing serum prostate-specific antigen (PSA) levels and androgen-independent growth.

Improved control over progression to androgen-independence may be accomplished by intermittent hormonal therapy. Foulds [2] and Noble [3] postulated that the replacement of androgens, even in small amounts, would have a conditioning effect on surviving cells allowing them to conserve or regain desirable traits of differentiation, and implied that long periods of hormone deprivation accelerated progression towards autonomous growth. Subsequent demonstrations that consecutive episodes of testosterone-induced regeneration of involuted prostate completely restored the susceptibility of the epithelium to further androgen withdrawal was an incentive to try simi-

KARGER

Fax + 41 61 306 12 34
E-Mail karger@karger.ch
www.karger.com

0302–2838/98/0349–0037$15.00/0

Accessible online at:
http://BioMedNet.com/karger

Dr. M. Gleave
D-9, 2733 Heather Street, Vancouver General Hospital
Vancouver, B.C. V5Z 3J5 (Canada)
Tel. +1 604 875 5003, Fax +1 604 875 5604
E-Mail gleave@unixg.ubc.ca

lar experiments on tumours. The underlying assumption was that the maintenance of apoptotic potential by successive rounds of androgen withdrawal and replacement (intermittent androgen suppression, IAS) might delay tumour progression.

However, IAS is a feasible treatment option only if immediate hormone therapy (i.e. at the time of diagnosis of metastatic or recurrent disease) is superior to delayed therapy (i.e. waiting for the development of symptoms). In this respect, accumulating evidence suggests that treatment should commence at the time of diagnosis of locally advanced or metastatic disease [4–6]. For example, in the Medical Research Council's study of 938 patients, progression from M0 to M1 disease and the development of metastatic pain occurred significantly more quickly in the delayed therapy group compared with the immediate therapy group [5].

With earlier diagnosis of prostate cancer now possible, patients presenting for the first time generally are younger, have an earlier disease stage and are expected to live longer. IAS may improve their quality of life by having the benefits of immediate androgen ablation while reducing therapy-induced side effects and costs.

Mechanisms of Progression to Androgen Independence

Cellular and molecular mechanisms that help mediate progression to androgen independence include expansion of pre-existing clones of androgen-independent cells (clonal selection), up-regulation of androgen-repressed adaptive mechanisms capable of aborting the apoptotic process (adaptation), androgen receptor mutations leading to a constitutively active transcriptional factor, or production of factors capable of interacting with the androgen receptor (protein-protein interactions) [7–9]. All are probably contributory factors to androgen independence in heterogeneous tumours such as prostate cancer. Clonal expansion of androgen-independent cells after castration cannot be prevented by current therapeutic strategies because of resistance to traditional cytotoxic chemotherapies. However, it may be possible to inhibit or modulate the adaptive changes in gene expression precipitated by androgen ablation through the differentiating influence of androgen.

The ability of benign or malignant prostate cells to undergo apoptosis and express PSA are acquired as a feature of differentiation of prostatic cells under the influence of androgens. Therefore, in the absence of androgens dividing cells cannot differentiate and become preapoptotic again; this explains why recurrent tumour growth after castration is characterized by androgen independence. Progression to androgen independence is, in part, directed by epigenetic factors (androgen ablation) and, as such, these factors may be a primary but quiescent property of some prostate cancer cells which are activated in response to androgen ablation. IAS is based on the hypothesis that if tumour cells that survive androgen withdrawal are forced into a normal pathway of differentiation by androgen replacement, then apoptotic potential might be restored and progression to androgen independence delayed. It follows that if androgens are replaced soon after regression of tumour, it should be possible to bring about repeated cycles of androgen-stimulated growth, differentiation, and regression of tumour in response to androgen ablation. IAS appears to prolong the time to development of androgen independence in both the Shionogi [10] and LNCaP [11] tumour models, providing preclinical evidence to support its testing in men with prostate cancer.

Clinical Studies of Intermittent Androgen Suppression

The intermittent regulation of serum testosterone levels was first attempted in 19 patients with advanced prostate cancer [12]. Patients received diethylstilboestrol (DES) until a clinical response was clearly demonstrated and then treatment was withheld until symptoms recurred. An improved quality of life was achieved owing to the reduced intake of DES, and no adverse effects on survival were apparent.

The development of a safe, reversible form of medical castration enables IAS, and serial serum PSA concentration measurements permit accurate monitoring of disease activity and serve as trigger points for stopping and restarting therapy. Preliminary results of IAS in 47 patients using reversible medical castration and serum PSA as trigger points were reported by Goldenberg et al. [13] and updated by Gleave et al. [14] (table 1). A total of 70 patients with a minimum follow-up of 12 months (mean 46 months) have now been accrued, 41 with clinically localized and 29 with metastatic disease. Treatment was initiated with combined androgen blockade and continued for an average of 9 months. Medication was then withheld until serum PSA increased to 10–20 ng/ml. This cycle of treatment and no treatment was repeated until the regulation of PSA became androgen independent (fig. 1).

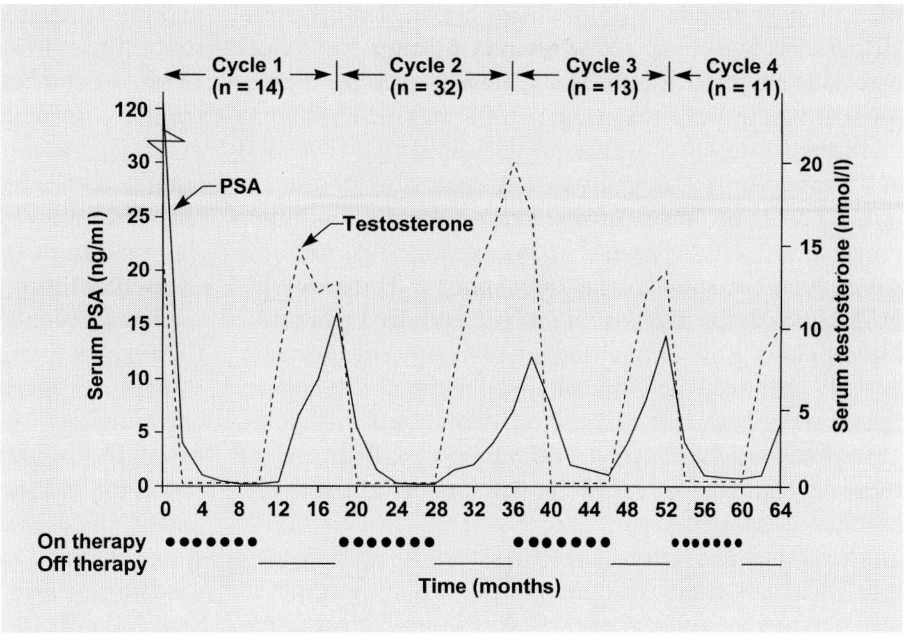

Fig. 1. Composite results from 70 patients treated for more than 1 year on an intermittent androgen suppression protocol, of whom 14 are in their 1st cycle of treatment, 32 in their 2nd cycle, 13 in their 3rd cycle, 5 in their 4th cycle, and 6 in their 5th cycle [13]. Mean serum PSA at the start of the 1st, 2nd, 3rd and 4th cycles was 110 ng/ml, 16 ng/ml, 12 ng/ml, and 14 ng/ml, respectively. The first 3 cycles averaged 18, 18, and 15.5 months in length, respectively, with on average 45% of time spent 'off' therapy. Adapted with permission [13].

Table 1. Clinical studies of intermittent androgen suppression

Investigator	Clinical stage	Mean follow-up months	PSA (ng/ml) at start (no. patients)			Mean cycle length (months; 1, 2, 3)	Time 'off' therapy, %	Mean time to nadir PSA (months)
			cycle 1	cycle 2	cycle 3			
Goldenberg [13]	Local + metastatic	30	128 (47)	15 (30)	18 (15)	18, 18, 16	47	5
Gleave [14]	Local + metastatic	46	110 (70)	16 (56)	12 (24)	18, 18, 16	47	5
Higano [15]	Local + metastatic	26	25 (22)	7.7 (12)	NA (0)	15, 18	38	3.5
Oliver [16]	Local + metastatic	NA	NA (20)	NA	NA	NA	NA	NA
Grossfield [17]	Local	24	21 (47)	7.0 (17)	20.5 (3)	16, 11, NA*	50	4*

* Treatment was continued for 1–2 months after nadir PSA was reached. NA, not available.

The 'off' treatment period in all cycles was associated with an improvement in sense of well-being, and the recovery of libido and potency in the men who reported normal or near-normal sexual function before the start of therapy. Androgen-independent progression occurred in 10 of 29 stage D patients and 7 of 41 patients with localized disease after a mean follow-up of 43 months. Of 21 stage D2 patients, 12 remain in the study with stable disease. Nine patients have died, three from non-cancer related illness; the median time to progression and overall survival of these patients was 26 and 42 months, respectively.

Since these initial reports, other investigators have confirmed the feasibility of IAS in patients with advanced or recurrent prostate cancer (table 1). Higano et al. [15] reported results from a cohort of 22 patients (7 stage D2, 3 stage D1, 2 stage T2–3, and 10 biochemical failures after definitive local therapy). All patients remain alive with two patients (1 biochemical relapse and 1 D1) progressing to androgen independence at 33 and 22 months, respectively. Time 'off' therapy for stage D2 patients was 35%, slightly less than the percentage of time 'off' therapy for biochemical relapsers (44%). All patients who were cycled 'off' therapy for 3 months or more noted some improvement in overall quality of life. Oliver et al. [16] reviewed 20 patients with localized or metastatic prostate cancer who elected to stop androgen ablation therapy after a median of 12 months (range 3–48 months). After a median of 9 months off therapy, 13 patients progressed and were restarted on androgen ablation, and 10 of these remain progression free after 2 years. Of particular interest because of the relatively long periods 'off' therapy, were seven patients who were 'on' then 'off' therapy for 3/33, 3/36, 3/43, 5/40, 12/36, 12/42 and 16/36 months. Grossfield et al. [17] reported on their initial experience with 47 patients with clinically localized prostate cancer. On average, patients completed two treatment cycles. Only one patient failed to respond to reinstitution of treatment, and no patients demonstrated progression during the follow-up period.

Observations from each of these small series suggest that relatively short 'on' therapy periods may result in 'off' therapy periods of several years, and implies that continuous therapy may represent over-treatment in a significant proportion of men. Some differences in treatment protocol deserve comment, particularly regarding potential candidates, and trigger points for stopping and restarting androgen withdrawal therapy.

Candidates and Trigger Points for Intermittent Androgen Suppression

Men with TXN1-3M0 or TXNXM1 who are sexually active, compliant to close follow-up, or who do not tolerate the side effects of androgen ablation can be considered for IAS as long as they understand that IAS is investigational. In addition, IAS should not be offered to patients who fail to reach serum PSA nadirs below 4 ng/ml after 6 months of therapy because of the associated short duration of response and poor prognosis [18]. We agree with Grossfield et al. [17] that biochemical failures after radiotherapy or surgery are groups most likely to benefit from IAS, when the benefits, costs and side effects of immediate therapy are taken into account.

Each 'on' treatment period should be continued until maximal castration-induced apoptosis and tumour regression has been induced, but stopped before constitutive development of the androgen-independent phenotype. We use a 9-month 'on' treatment period because PSA nadir and maximal soft tissue regression is not reached until 8–9 months in many patients [14]. Premature termination of therapy would permit some cancer cells destined to undergo apoptosis to survive upon reexposure to testosterone. Some investigators treat for 1–2 months past PSA nadir for each individual patient, which results in shorter 'on' cycles and shorter 'off' cycles, but similar percentages of time spent 'off' therapy [18]. However, the definition of nadir must be consistent, and should be the lowest plateau serum PSA concentration attained following institution of androgen ablation. Standardization of treatment regimens is necessary for comparison of future series.

Trigger points for reinstitution of androgen withdrawal therapy were similar among investigators [13–17]. Although the optimal time remains undefined and empirical, time 'off' therapy should be long enough to permit normalization of testosterone-induced tumour cell differentiation and improved quality of life. Trigger points are usually individualized for each patient and factors that are considered include PSA levels before treatment, disease stage, PSA velocity, presence of symptoms, and tolerance of androgen ablation therapy. In general, in patients with metastatic disease and high pre-treatment PSA levels, therapy is restarted when PSA concentration increases to 20 ng/ml. In patients with locally recurrent disease and moderately elevated pre-treatment PSA levels, therapy is restarted when PSA concentration reaches 6–15 ng/ml, and earlier for post-radical prostatectomy recurrences.

It is important to look for other signs of progressive disease when serum PSA is used to monitor disease activity, in case of the unusual scenario of PSA-negative disease progression. The outcome of IAS may be improved by increasing the length and number of cycles. Prolongation of each 'off' treatment period may be possible (e.g. with 5-α-reductase inhibitors) and of 'on' treatment periods by apoptotic-enhancing agents (e.g. using antisense Bcl-2 strategies), differentiating agents, or gene therapies at specific times during a cycle of treatment.

Conclusion

Observations from accumulating experience in phase II studies suggest that IAS is a feasible treatment option which improves quality of life and does not appear to have a negative impact on time to progression or survival. However, whether survival is affected in a positive or negative fashion remains unknown and can only be answered by phase III randomized studies which are now being initiated in several countries.

References

1 Denis L, Murphy GP: Overview of phase III trials on combined androgen treatment in patients with metastatic prostate cancer. Cancer 1993;72(suppl):3888–3895.
2 Foulds L: Neoplastic Development 1. New York, Academic Press, 1969.
3 Noble RL: Hormonal control of growth and progression in tumors of Nb rats and a theory of action. Cancer Res 1977;37:82–94.
4 Byar DP: Proceedings: The Veterans Administration Cooperative Urological Research Group's studies of cancer of the prostate. Cancer 1973;32:1126–1130.
5 The Medical Research Council Prostate Cancer Working Party Investigators Group: Immediate vs deferred treatment for advanced prostate cancer: Initial results of the MRC trial. Br J Urol 1997;79:235–246.
6 Bolla M, Gonzalez D, Warde P, Dubois JB, Mirimanoff R-O, Storme G, Bernier J, Kuten A, Sternberg C, Gil T, Colette L, Pierart M: Improved survival in patients with locally advanced prostate cancer treated with radiotherapy and goserelin. N Engl J Med 1997;337:295–300.
7 Bruchovsky N, Brown EM, Coppin CM, Goldenberg SL, LeRiche JC, Murray NC, Rennie PS: The endocrinology and treatment of prostate tumor progression. Prog Clin Biol Res 1987;239:348–387.
8 Isaacs JT, Wake N, Coffey DS, Sandberg AA: Genetic instability coupled to clonal selection as a mechanism for progression in prostatic cancer. Cancer Res 1982;42:2353–2361.
9 Gleave ME, Hsieh JT: Experimental animal models for prostate cancer; in Lange P, Scher H, and Ragavahn O (eds): Genitourinary Oncology. Lippincott, 1997, pp 367–378.
10 Akakura K, Bruchovsky N, Goldenberg SL, Rennie PS, Buckley AR, Sullivan LD: Effects of intermittent androgen suppression on androgen-dependent tumours: apoptosis and serum prostate specific antigen. Cancer 1993;71: 2782–2790.
11 Sato N, Gleave ME, Bruchovsky N, Goldenberg SL, Rennie P, Sullivan LD: Intermittent androgen suppression delays time to non-androgen regulated prostate specific antigen gene expression in the human prostate LNCaP tumour model. J Steroid Biochem Mol Biol 1996; 58:139–146.
12 Klotz LH, Herr HW, Morse MJ, Whitmore WF Jr: Intermittent endocrine therapy for advanced prostate cancer. Cancer 1986;58:2546–2250.
13 Goldenberg SL, Bruchovsky N, Gleave ME, Sullivan LD, Akakura K: Intermittent androgen suppression in the treatment of prostate cancer: A preliminary report. Urology 1995;45: 839–845.
14 Gleave ME, Bruchovsky N, Goldenberg SL, Rennie P: Intermittent androgen suppression: rationale and clinical experience; in Schröder F (ed): Recent Advances in Prostate Cancer and BPH. London, Parthenon, 1997, pp 109–121.
15 Higano CS, Ellis W, Russell K, Lange PH: Intermittent androgen suppression with leuprolide and flutamide for prostate cancer. A pilot study. Urology 1996;48:800–804.
16 Oliver RT, Williams G, Paris AM, Blandy JP: Intermittent androgen deprivation after PSA-complete response as a strategy to reduce induction of hormone-resistant prostate cancer. Urology 1997;49:79–82.
17 Grossfield GD, Small EJ, Carrol PR: Intermittent androgen deprivation for clinically localized prostate cancer: initial experience. Urology 1998;51:137–144.
18 Miller JI, Ahmann FR, Drach GW, Emerson SS, Bottaccini MR: The clinical usefulness of serum prostate specific antigen after hormonal therapy of metastatic prostate cancer. J Urol 1992;147:956–961.

European
Urology

D. Newling[a]
F. Debruyne[b]

Conclusion

[a] Department of Urology, Academic Hospital Vrije University, Amsterdam;
[b] Department of Urology, University Hospital Nijmegen, The Netherlands

The symposium 'The management of prostate cancer in the third millennium' and the workshop 'Therapeutic dilemmas in prostate cancer' at the XIIIth Congress of the European Association of Urology 1998 in Barcelona both highlighted that there are many questions and outstanding issues surrounding the management of prostate cancer that need to be addressed. Nevertheless, we now understand more of the mechanisms underlying the disease process, and results from clinical studies are providing us with more information on which to base treatment strategies.

During the workshop, two case histories were described and discussed among the faculty, and the delegates voted on which treatment option they would have recommended. This gave an interesting insight into the preferred treatments of this international audience which was made even more interesting by a comparison of votes on the first case history with those obtained at the XIIth Congress of the European Association of Urology in Paris, September 1–5, 1996.

Case History 1

In the first case, provided by Dr Hartwig Huland, Germany, a 50-year-old man went to a urologist for a routine check-up. A small (1 cm) node was detected in the right prostate lobe which was surrounded by benign prostatic enlargement. His serum prostate-specific antigen (PSA) concentration was 6.8 ng/ml, and he had a transrectal ultrasound of 42 g, benign prostatic hyperplasia (BPH) with a hypodense area in the peripheral zone on the right lobe. His residual urine was less than 10 ml. After ultrasound-guided systemic biopsies, two of the biopsies from the right lobe were positive with a Gleason score of 3+3. No cancer was detected in the biopsy of the right base and in the biopsy taken from the left side. A bone scan was negative. Most of the audience (49%) said that their preferred therapy was radical retropubic prostatectomy with unilateral nerve sparing, and a significant proportion (23%) voted for radical retropubic prostatectomy with bilateral nerve sparing. These results were very similar to those obtained in Paris (45% and 26%, respectively).

The patient in fact underwent bilateral lymphadenectomy of the obturator node and radical retropubic prostatectomy with unilateral nerve sparing on the left side. A specimen showed a pT3aN0M0 Gleason 3+4 with capsular penetration on the right side with a positive margin. The patient recovered well, achieving normal micturition and perfect continence within a few weeks. At this stage watchful waiting as a treatment strategy was chosen by 50% of the audience in Barcelona, and 33% opted for postoperative radiotherapy because it was a pT3 tumour with a positive margin. Again these results were similar to those from Paris although slightly fewer voted for watchful waiting in Paris (44%) and more voted for hormonal treatment (20% versus only 6% in Barcelona). The patient's illness was managed by watchful waiting and he remained asymptomatic.

The PSA concentration remained unmeasurable for the next 3 years, after which it became slightly raised with a slow doubling time (rising to 0.6, 0.9, and 1.8 ng/ml during 1 year). The audience was divided at this stage over what they would do: 27% chose watchful waiting, 25%

KARGER
Fax +41 61 306 12 34
E-Mail karger@karger.ch
www.karger.com

0302–2838/98/0349–0042$15.00/0

Accessible online at:
http://BioMedNet.com/karger

Prof. Don Newling, Academic Hospital Vrije University, Polikliniek Urologie, PO Box 7057
NL–0117 MB Amsterdam (The Netherlands), Tel. +31 204 440272, Fax + 31 206 425085
Prof. Frans Debruyne, 426 Department of Urology, University Hospital Nijmegen
Geert Grootplein 10, PO Box 9101, NL–6500 HB Nijmegen (The Netherlands)
Tel. + 31 243 613735, Fax + 31 243 541031

local radiotherapy, 20% local biopsy and 17% hormonal therapy. This had also been true of the audience in Paris although slightly more people had voted for local radiotherapy (35%) and hormonal therapy (28%) with fewer voting for watchful waiting (23%) and local biopsy (13%). In reality, the patient elected for watchful waiting but a local biopsy revealed prostate cancer in the area of the prostatectomy. The patient underwent local radiotherapy after which serum PSA concentration was reduced from 2.3 ng/ml to less than 0.4 ng/ml.

Case History 2

In the second case history, from Frans Debruyne, comparative votes with the meeting in Paris were not available. However, the exercise still revealed an interesting insight into treatment choices being made by clinicians. The patient was a 53-year-old man who had presented with progressive obstructive complaints over 4 years. Investigations revealed a 2 cm indurated region, palpable in the right prostate lobe by digital rectal examination (DRE). This was surrounded by benign prostatic enlargement which was judged to be 36 g by ultrasound. A transrectal biopsy showed a Gleason score of 6, the patient's serum PSA concentration was 5 ng/ml and the stage of the tumour was T2N0M0. An overwhelming majority of the audience (71%) thought that the cancer should be managed with a radical retropubic prostatectomy, with the second choice being a radical retropubic prostatectomy after 3 months' neoadjuvant treatment (voted for by 13% of the audience). The patient had insisted on neoadjuvant treatment with combined androgen blockade (CAB) which consisted of a luteinizing hormone-releasing hormone (LH-RH) agonist plus a non-steroidal antiandrogen.

DRE revealed no further abnormalities after 3 months' neoadjuvant treatment and the size of the prostate was reduced by more than 60%. At this point most of the audience (73%) thought that radical retropubic prostatectomy should be performed and, indeed, the patient did opt for a limited lymphadenectomy and a radical retropubic prostatectomy. The pathological evaluation of the cancer was pT2N0M0, Gleason score 7. The patient remained asymptomatic and regained normal micturition and continence. PSA remained undetectable for more than 2 years after which the serum concentration rose to 1.7 ng/ml; there were no abnormalities detected by DRE. At this stage, 41% of the audience thought that watchful waiting should be employed and the second choice was local radiotherapy (31%). Watchful waiting was in fact chosen and the patient remained asymptomatic, although PSA concentrations slowly increased (by 0.8 ng/ml in the first year and by 0.6 ng/ml in the second year).

Four years after surgery there was a sharper increase in serum PSA concentration to a level of 6.5 ng/ml. There was a dubious induration detected by DRE but a biopsy was negative. After a further 6 months PSA concentration had risen to 9.9 ng/ml, there was a local recurrence and Gleason score of 7 but no complaints from the patient. Many in the audience thought that local radiotherapy (46%) or CAB therapy (32%) would be a good treatment strategy. However, the patient had been reluctant to undergo treatment while he was asymptomatic. As the patient's serum PSA concentration increased by 4 ng/ml over the subsequent 6 months, the patient consented to a bone scan which was negative and a CT scan which showed para-iliac lymph node enlargement on the right side. Knowing this, 55% of the audience thought that CAB would be the best treatment option and this is also what the patient chose.

After 1 month of treatment, serum PSA was undetectable. The audience was divided at this point between recommending to continue CAB (40%) or trying intermittent hormonal treatment (54%). The patient was happy to continue CAB; after 1 year he switched to a combination of an antiandrogen and 5-α-reductase inhibitor in the hope of reducing further loss of potency and libido. After receiving a further year of treatment, his PSA concentration increased from 0.3 ng/ml to 3.6 ng/ml in a 6-month period. The majority of the audience (72%) at this stage thought that the treatment should be switched back to a combination of LH-RH agonist plus antiandrogen and this is what happened. Initially there was a decrease in serum PSA concentration but after 9 months it began to rise rapidly. Diffuse bone metastases were seen on a bone scan and X-ray, and there was a rapid progression of the tumour and hormone resistance developed. At this stage 45% of the audience thought that it would be best to stop antiandrogen treatment and 30% of the audience recommended treatment with strontium 90.

Discussion

As well as providing an interesting insight into varying opinions on the best way to manage prostate cancer, these case histories also illustrated the point that clinicians face many different situations, even in the treatment of one patient. The treatment choice depends very much on the

stage of disease, age of the patient, and particular wishes of the patient. In a set of more general questions, 59% of the audience thought that they would be able to offer definitive therapeutic advice to a patient with early prostate cancer, 23% were not sure and 14% would not be able to offer definitive advice. With a patient who has histologically confirmed prostate cancer which is judged operable, most of the audience (84%) said that their advice would take into account the age of the patient rather than the grade of tumour. Patients vary in the level of symptoms that they consider acceptable, the audience in Barcelona also differed on the level of incontinence or impotence they considered acceptable in exchange for a cure for early prostate cancer by radical therapy; 55% of the audience would advocate 5% incontinence although 21% of the audience felt that a 20% incontinence rate after radical prostatectomy was acceptable. For impotence, 51% of the audience accepted an impotence rate of 60%, although 20% of the audience thought 40% or 100% was acceptable.

Conclusion

Many of the speakers at the symposium and workshop stressed the need for further research on the best way to manage prostate cancer. This should go hand in hand with basic research which would clarify the mechanisms involved and help to develop markers for disease progression. We always hope for a rational approach to treating disease and for a better prognosis to offer the patient. Some of the approaches that remain experimental at this point, such as intermittent hormonal therapy, may do much to improve patients' survival and quality of life if they are established as effective therapies. After listening to the presentations at the XIIIth Congress of the European Association of Urology 1998 we have every reason to be optimistic about the treatment of prostate cancer as we approach the new millennium.